The 3:00 PM SECRET

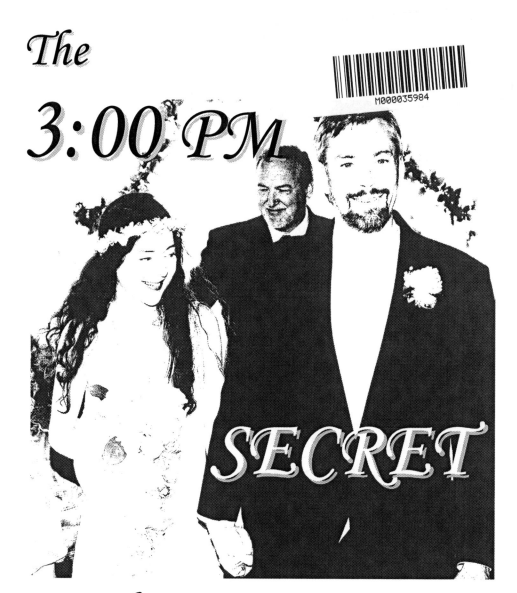

Live Slim and Strong
Live Your Dreams

Including A Man's Perspective

Debra Anne Ross Lawrence

GlacierDog Publishing

A Division of GlacierDog Intergalactica

~ *The 3:00 PM SECRET* ~
Live Slim and Strong
Live Your Dreams

Notice To The Reader

The author and publisher have done their best to present accurate and up-to-date information in this book, but cannot guarantee that the information is correct or will suit your particular situation. If you do anything recommended in this book without the supervision of a licensed medical doctor or other appropriate professional advisor, you do so at your own risk. The author and publisher present this information for educational purposes only, and do not attempt to prescribe any medical treatment. If you require expert assistance, you should obtain this assistance from a competent professional.

TABLE OF CONTENTS

Isn't it ironic that *diet* books are all about *food?*

Why focus on the very thing you are trying to avoid?

Dieting fills the mind with buying, preparing, and eating certain *foods.*

Food becomes an end in itself - the center of a food-focused life.

Food is merely a source of nutrition and energy, not a life purpose.

How can you be slim and strong if your life revolves around your next meal?

Free yourself from a food-focused life - and rediscover your *dreams.*

A slim and strong body makes living your *dreams* possible.

Find your purpose and destiny - live your *dreams.*

Prologue

A Man's Perspective

ASKING "WHY?"

"But we've always done it this way." A company refusing to re-examine its basic practices and to adapt is doomed. "Don't trust anyone over 30." Boomers took pride in questioning their parents' values, politics, and faith, asking foundational questions, but were less skeptical and rebellious about nutritional values and faith in processed foods. As functioning adults we are able to think for ourselves, but have we inherited and adopted unhealthy practices from our ancestors without examining them critically? If today we and our families were truly healthy and fit, complacency may be justified, but we are not. We're wasting millions treating symptoms of poor lifestyle choices rather than uprooting the causes.

AM I "OK"?

I was slow to begin questioning the health and nutrition practices of my youth. My parents meant well, and were often frustrated when I refused many good foods that I didn't "like". I learned to eat three meals a day, with the big meal in the evening. At breakfast I put sugar on my corn flakes, ate "squishy bread" toast with butter, and downed a pastry. My lunch box always included chips and a cookie. Dinners invariably offered meat, starch, and a sweet dessert. We had evening snacks, often soft drinks or sweets near bedtime. Since candy was available, efforts to limit my intake met limited success. Daily exercise was not modeled, though fortuitously I loved so many sports and games I burned off my abundant calories and stayed fit. Like most kids, I watched too much television and loved to stay up late.

As an adult, I kept up the exercise despite a desk job, so I never carried more than an extra 10 to 20 pounds. The old practices, however, stayed with me, and I knew that I was not optimizing my health and longevity. The extra weight kept me from top performance in my running, skiing, climbing, and similar activities. My diet had improved since my youth, but I still ate and snacked too much, consuming food with poor nutritional value and too much harmful content. While I knew that today's foods lack the nutritional content of foods of the past, and I was suspicious of pesticides and growth hormones, the thought of migrating to an organic, vegetarian, unprocessed food lifestyle seemed extreme. After all, could all those chefs, grocery stores, and food companies be wrong?

TOO "RADICAL"?

I probably would not have made "radical" changes (I never was much of a radical) unless inspired and strongly encouraged by the author. Frankly, the changes were not really radical at all in an extremist sense of the word, though they were significantly different in key ways from my traditional practices. To a person accustomed to the book's recommendations, my *former* practices would seem truly radical, even foolhardy. Further, if you are one of the many who have repeatedly tried and failed to achieve the fit and healthy body you want, you are probably open to a few fundamental and major (i.e. "radical") improvements to you daily routine!

TIME TO "DECIDE"?

For years I had many inklings that I needed to break away from my destructive practices, but needed outside help to tip the balance and start me on a new path. I was partially persuaded to follow this path by the solid research findings that point the way, and the logic behind the ideas. I also was persuaded at a deeper level by the living testimony of our author, who began changing her lifestyle over a decade ago toward the methods shared in her book. She experienced a great resurgence of health, a beautifully "young" and fit body, and the freedom to pursue her dreams. There also was a very practical consideration: It is ideal for people sharing a life together to maintain similar and compatible eating, sleeping, and exercise practices. So I finally put aside excuses and decided to reconstruct these aspects of my life.

RESULTS?

At the time of this writing, I have followed the author's recommendations for about 18 months (sometimes with greater fidelity than the author herself!). I have benefited tremendously from implementing these changes to my eating and sleeping habits (I didn't need to increase my exercise). First, I disposed of 15 useless pounds to within 5 pounds of my ideal, and stayed there even through holidays. I look and feel younger, and my mind is sharper. I have been in nearly perfect health. I spend less time preparing food and cleaning up the kitchen, and now realize how uncomfortable it feels to go to bed on a full stomach. Importantly, I have greater confidence and peace of mind now that I am helping my body avoid deterioration and myriads of diseases by properly nourishing my organs and systems, saving them from infusions of toxic chemicals and harmful "foods." These many improvements, though, seem like mere fringe benefits to marrying the author who is very interesting and inspiring even when **not** exhorting me or donning her lab coat! Our plans for a long life together include adventures requiring health and vigor!

WHAT ABOUT YOU AND YOURS?

Undoubtedly most "diet" and health books are purchased by women, though the men and children in their lives have the same health needs and desires. It may be as difficult to eat nutritionally in a house full of junk food addicts as it is to stop smoking in a family of smokers. It's hard to add exercise to the daily routine while surrounded by "inertia experts," and almost impossible to go to sleep early with "night owls" hooting. If you want to implement the beneficial changes discussed in this book, you will be more successful if you bring your family and also a few friends along with you. Isn't it just as important for them to take the same life-enhancing and possibly life-saving steps so they can last as long and keep up with you?

For these reasons, please don't keep the "Secret" or presume the book's principles are appropriate only for women. The themes may appeal more to women because they may care more about their health and appearance, but you women can appeal to the men and children in your lives to care more about their own health and appearance because you love them. The author's message and mission are appropriate for everyone seriously seeking a long, healthy, active life!

David Allen Lawrence

Discover Your Destiny

Decide To Be Slim and Strong

Eat Early Each Day

Follow the Ten Nutrition Tips

Enjoy a Ten-Minute Daily Workout

Give Yourself Generous Sleep

Live your Dreams

Acknowledgements

I began developing and practicing the tenets described in this book in the early 1990's, and began seriously researching and writing the book in 1998. During the ensuing 9-year period I researched, revised, and fine tuned the text in order to create a book that clearly describes the philosophy and practical steps that can secure and maintain a trim, fit body, and set you on the path to realizing your dreams.

Since the inception of my work on this book, my mother, Maggie Ross, has been a tireless and trustworthy sounding board and source of support, encouragement, and sagacious comments. She has read and commented on the manuscript countless times. I am grateful for her time, wisdom, photography, and excellent editing skills.

My sister, Jan Ross, MSW, was an early reviewer of the manuscript, and I appreciate the many useful comments she provided. My wonderful friends, Kathy Williams and Connie Baer, R.N., also read an early version of the manuscript, and I am grateful for the helpful feedback they each provided. I especially thank the Certified Physical Trainer in California who reviewed and provided guidance on the exercise positions and instructions. I am also indebted to Dr. Arlene Giordano for carefully reading an early version of the manuscript and for her valuable comments and suggestions.

I am particularly grateful to my mentor and friend Professor Channing Robertson for his careful reading and numerous invaluable comments and suggestions on the manuscript. I also sincerely appreciate his gracious and generous endorsement.

Finally, I am eternally grateful to my brilliant and beautiful husband, David Allen Lawrence, for carefully reading and editing the manuscript multiple times, making innumerable perspicacious comments and suggestions, helping amplify the motivational aspects of the message, providing enthusiastic and practical support of my efforts to complete and publish the book, helping me finalize the cover and navigate the publishing process, generously endorsing the book, and sharing his personal testimony in the prologue "A Man's Perspective".

Preview

"Hello?" said Sandy, wondering who would be calling her so late.

"It's Isabelle. I'm in Tahiti!" squealed her friend.

"Wow! What are you doing there? I mean ... that's great!" Sandy stammered in surprise.

"I'm rewarding myself. I finally lost weight. I reached my goal! So I booked a flight, and here I am! Just like that! The ocean is sparkling. It's beautiful!" shrieked Isabelle.

"Wow! I think I hear the call of some exotic bird coming through the phone. So ... how did you do it?" Sandy asked, as she stared at her caramel popcorn and mini-doughnut decorated coffee table.

"Do what?" Isabelle said.

"Lose all that weight," said Sandy.

"It was so easy. I'll never be fat again!" said a triumphant Isabelle.

"But how?" Sandy pressed.

"I found a book called 'The 3:00 PM Secret: Live Slim and Strong, Live Your Dreams'. I just made the adjustments it recommended. It gave me back my dreams."

"Will you go back to Tahiti with me after I get the book and reach my goal?" asked Sandy hopefully.

"You better believe it!" said Isabelle.

We all know that if we consistently restrict calories, eat nutritiously, and exercise an hour or more each day, we could eventually achieve our desired weight and feel better. If this was easy to do, most people would resemble athletes and models, and obesity would not be epidemic. The difficulty in controlling weight over time is living a life of endless discipline, denial, and deprivation. *The 3:00 PM Secret* offers a better, achievable solution.

Have you tried to achieve your ideal body, but the prospect of never-ending self-denial and endless restrictive eating was too depressing to seriously contemplate? Have you tried and failed too many times to count? Are you at the end of your rope in frustration and despair over your inability to control your weight? If so, you can achieve permanent weight-control success by adopting a rhythm of *3:00 PM days* and *Free days*. (See Chapter 2.)

Do your dieting practices weaken your body through inadequate nutrition so that you crave unnecessary calories as your body tries to get the nutrients it needs? If you follow the *Ten Tips For Good Nutrition,* they will help you control your weight and be healthier without craving too much food. (See Chapter 3 and Appendix 1.)

Do you want to exercise thirty to sixty minutes a day, but never find time? Do you have no real desire to exercise at all? Given the numerous health and weight control benefits, could you dedicate just ten minutes a day? The quick, easy, convenient, muscle-building *ten-minute maximized workout* is a great way to get consistent and effective daily exercise. (See Chapter 4.)

Do you often eat because you are tired and want energy even though you're not really hungry? Do you eat more than you need "just to get through the day"? Eating for the energy you should be getting from sleep can sabotage your weight control efforts. Don't eat because you are tired – learn why getting adequate sleep can help you lose weight and be healthier. (See Chapter 5.)

Most importantly, are you really living the life you have always dreamed about? Do you want to spend your life wishing you looked and felt better so you could pursue those dreams? Can you take your focus off food and embark on your true life's journey? You must *decide* how you truly want to spend the rest of your life, and if you want it to be in a body that will support your aspirations. (See Chapter 1.)

The *3:00 PM Secret*, if integrated into your life, will become second nature, and will not only keep you trim and fit, but will also improve your chances of successful aging. Chapter 6, *Successful Aging*, discusses encouraging research on aging and the benefits of applying many of the same principles used for weight control to living a longer, healthier, happier life. Our ability to affect our own lifespan, as well as our physical and mental aging process, can motivate us to make an ideal body and sharp mind a reality.

Before beginning to practice the *3:00 PM Secret* lifestyle described in the following pages, please read the "How To Begin" cut-out section at the end of this book. Also, at the end of this book are cut-out pages of the "Daily Workout Summary" exercises. In addition, please see the website for this book: www.ThreePMSecret.com.

Chapter 1

The Decision

"So what finally motivated you to get serious and lose weight?" Sandy's questions could not await Isabelle's return from Tahiti.

"Oh, Sandy, I just couldn't take it anymore! I was so unhappy with my life and my body. I was so bored with my job – you know I always wanted to be a geologist, but somehow ended up in accounting. I was 'practical' and took the easy route. I was afraid to follow my dreams." Isabelle thought of her wasted years as she looked out her hotel window at the ocean, which seemed to glisten like the new life she was anticipating.

"Isabelle, I never realized you had been so unhappy. Then what?"

*"One day I was wandering around a little bookstore and there it was – The 3:00 PM Secret book. I began reading it, and it seemed to speak to my soul. It said **I** had to make a **decision**, which I was **so** ready to do! That ingenious eating style of the 3:00 PM days really appealed to me. The doable ten-minute workout made sense, and the idea of giving myself permission to get the sleep I knew I needed was a relief. It totally resonated with me. Sandy, as I read more later that night I decided to get my life together, to honor the body God gave me, and to be free to do what my heart told me was my real life purpose, my destiny. That was it – I began my new journey."*

"And you're celebrating it in Tahiti. You've inspired me, Isabelle."

In the beginning of the first book of the Mrs. Pollifax series by Dorothy Gilman, Mrs. Pollifax, a widow, is in her doctor's office. The doctor tells Mrs. Pollifax that she is in excellent physical health, however, he detects signs of depression. Mrs. Pollifax, in fact, feels she has no real purpose in her life, and that she has outlived her usefulness. The doctor asks her if there had ever been anything she longed to do but she had not had the time or freedom to pursue. On reflection, what floats into Mrs. Pollifax's mind is the shocking notion that she has always wanted to be a spy! Well, Mrs. Pollifax excitedly, but with trepidation, embarked upon her journey to become a spy, and the books describe her extraordinary adventures. What the doctor asked is something you need not wait to consider until you feel you have *"outlived your usefulness"*. You can begin today to think about and pursue whatever fascinates you and would bring meaning and adventure into your life. You can contemplate what is exciting and captivating, and take steps toward making it part of your life.

If you are not happy with your life, your dissatisfaction may be manifesting itself in the form of overeating or other self-destructive habits. Rather than surrendering to your situation, why not focus your attention instead on investigating what extraordinary new options exist for you? Even if you are already extremely busy, it is important to stop from time to time to reflect on your life's direction and consider what would give your life greater meaning. You could begin by asking yourself the *twenty-million dollar question*: "If I had twenty-million dollars in the bank and never had to work again, how would I spend my time for the rest of my life?" This question is not as easy to answer as it may seem. Contemplating this question holds many more exciting possibilities for how you may enhance your life rather than focusing your attention on eating (unless, of course, your dream is to become a chef). To get started, you could wander though a library or bookstore and look through books on various topics that have always seemed intriguing. What really captivates you and holds your attention? What were you put here to do? What do you think is God's purpose for your life? Test your ideas by looking through books and magazines on subjects you are drawn to and see if they hold your attention. You can also test ideas by talking to people who know you, as well as people knowledgeable in fields that interest you. As you discover what you feel passionate about, begin to reorder your life so you can be immersed in what you truly love and enjoy. Once you discover what captivates you, you can embark on a new journey, turning those interests into a life-long adventure.

Focusing mental energy on finding your purpose and making your dreams a reality will feed your soul, stimulate your brain, and keep your mind and body younger longer. At the same time, you will find yourself less passionate about eating and other potentially destructive activities. Even if you feel so overwhelmed with the day-to-day demands of your life and can't conceive of adding one more item to your schedule, give yourself the mental time to ask the fundamental questions about your life's purposes and passions. There is always mental time when you drive, shower, etc., to begin to reflect on what you may be replacing with food, and what might provide greater fulfillment.

Why live a life of unfulfilled dreams that you stuff down with food? Determine how you most want to spend the limited days of your life, and ***decide*** you are willing to do what it takes to make your wish a reality. Determine how you want your body to look and feel, and ***decide*** to do what it takes to make it what you want it to be. Every day time passes, and each day quickly becomes the past, lost forever. Every day brings us closer to the end of the year, the end of the decade, and the end of life. If you want to have the body and life you desire become a reality, but continually put off making it so, you will look back after years have passed and wonder where the time went and why you have not been living the way you really wanted to live. The truth is, the only person who can stop you from being exactly what you want to be and having the life you desire is you. Don't just wish your body was the way it was designed to be, ***decide to change it***. An analogy that demonstrates the difference between the concept of "I *wish*" and "I have *decided"* is: I wish I knew how to play the piano -versus- I have decided to learn to play the piano, and I am taking lessons once a week and practicing thirty minutes every day. There is a big difference between *wish* and ***decide***, and then *actually beginning*.

If you are reading this book, you are probably not satisfied with the image you are projecting to the world and to yourself. Can you deny that looking in the mirror and seeing a fit, healthy, and attractive person looking back at you would make you feel better? You may work diligently to achieve and accomplish certain goals, or spend hard-earned money on haircuts, clothing, and an education, and still feel hampered because you have not taken proper care of your body. If you are currently unhappy with your body's weight and condition, do you really want to go through the rest of this year and the rest of your life with the added physical and psychological burden of feeling unhealthy, always wishing you looked and felt better? Don't you want to live in a body that is easy to move around, and feels strong and capable? Do you want to be able to dress yourself every day without it being a monumental effort involving trying on multiple outfits until you find something that looks reasonably flattering? Do you want to feel stronger, healthier, and more empowered? There is nothing that can stop you from achieving the size, shape, and fitness level you want. It is entirely up to you.

Don't give up on living in your ideal body because of past failures in exercise and weight control. Don't be a permanent victim of fleeting whims that move you away from your goals. The principles described in this book provide a simple and achievable formula for permanent success. You only need to ***decide*** that you want to live your life at your desired weight and fitness level more than you want to cling to destructive habits and empty instant gratification. *The 3:00 PM Secret* allows you to gain and maintain a trim and fit body, and also have regular intervals of gratification so you can still enjoy life, go out to dinner, and relax with friends and family on the weekends.

An additional benefit of *The 3:00 PM Secret* is that it will always be available and work for you. Even if you get away from its guidelines for a period of time because of illness, vacation, or other disruptions in your life, you can always come back and get your body under control without endless, constant deprivation. If you follow *The 3:00 PM Secret*, you will have found a way to permanently control your weight and have the body that supports your aspirations.

After *deciding* you are willing to work toward your ideal body, you should determine exactly what *your* ideal body will look like. How do you truly want your body to look and feel? What do you think is your optimum weight range and fitness level? Do you merely want to look good in your clothes and have the basic strength to walk up three flights of stairs without getting winded, or do you want the finely tuned body of a ballet dancer, gymnast, or martial artist? This will depend on what you need your body to do, and the degree of physical strength you need in your life and future. We need our bodies to assist us in achieving the purpose and goals of life, not to be an unnecessary hindrance. How we look, dress, speak, and carry ourselves, as well as our perceived strength and capability, shapes how other people (who don't know us intimately) perceive and judge us, and often limits or expands the opportunities that may open up to us.

~~~

In case you still haven't made a **decision** to live in your ideal body, and are not sure you really want to control your weight, let me put on my lab coat and see if the following information tilts your thinking: Over two-thirds of U.S. adults are either overweight or obese.[1] Since the 1980's, the number of obese adults has nearly doubled. Excess weight and physical inactivity account for more than 300,000 premature deaths each year in the United States, second only to smoking-related deaths. People who are overweight or obese are more likely to develop heart disease, stroke, high blood pressure, diabetes, gallbladder disease, gout, sleep apnea, osteoarthritis, and certain types of cancer. High blood pressure, also called hypertension, is one of the leading causes of kidney failure. People with kidney failure must either endure dialysis or receive a kidney transplant to stay alive.[2] The American

---

[1] Science News v.165, No.9, p.139, 2/28/04

[2] http://kidney.niddk.nih.gov/kudiseases/pubs/highblood, NIDDK is part of the National Institutes of Health

Institute for Cancer Research concluded that obesity is consistently linked to post-menopausal breast cancer, colon cancer, endometrial cancer, prostate cancer, and kidney cancer.[3] As people get fatter, they become more susceptible to a host of chronic and life-threatening diseases, including diabetes, atherosclerosis, and cancer.

Why does obesity increase the risk of so many diseases? One link between increased disease and obesity is that certain cells (macrophage cells) usually associated with the immune system appear to move into fatty tissue. These macrophage cells seem to be a primary source of chemicals that spark inflammation in fat and elsewhere. There is increasing evidence that these inflammatory secretions from adipose tissue can foster disease.[4] One of these diseases, diabetes, is a progressive and serious illness involving complications such as kidney failure, heart disease, stroke, blindness, nerve damage, circulatory problems, wound healing problems often resulting in amputations, male impotence, and other debilitating health problems. Research studies and clinical trials have demonstrated that Type II diabetes can be largely prevented with a healthy diet and lifestyle, and that excess weight is the greatest risk factor for diabetes. Maintaining a healthy body weight and avoiding weight gain during adulthood is the cornerstone of diabetes prevention. Increasing physical activity and reducing sedentary behaviors such as prolonged television watching are also important factors in maintaining a healthy body weight and improving insulin sensitivity.[5] Still not convinced? Several studies have shown that people with Type II diabetes have twice the risk of developing Alzheimer's disease as non-diabetics.[6]

Researchers have also found that human fat cells produce a protein that is linked to both inflammation and an increased risk of heart disease and stroke. The protein, called C-reactive protein (CRP), is currently used diagnostically to predict future cardiovascular problems. The discovery that fat cells produce CRP may help explain why people who are overweight usually have higher levels of the molecule, and how body fat participates in vascular inflammation and the inflammatory processes that lead to cardiovascular disease.[7]

---

[3] U.S. Food and Drug administration, FDA Consumer magazine, January-February 2002

[4] Science News v.165, No.9, p.139, 2/28/04

[5] Annu Rev Public Health v.26, p.445, 2005

[6] Science v.301, No.5629, p.40, 7/4/03

[7] J Am Coll Cardiol, 2005; v.46, p.1112, 9/20/05online; http://www.medicalnewstoday.com/medicalnews.php?newsid=30761

A link between obesity and Alzheimer's disease was also shown in a study that revealed that women who are overweight (with a Body Mass Index of 29.3) at age 70 had an increased risk of developing Alzheimer's disease. See Appendix 2: Body Mass Index (BMI.) This study found that for every 1.0 unit increase in BMI at age 70 years, Alzheimer's disease risk increased by an astounding 36%.[8] Because so many of us are obese, and obesity continues to rise at an alarming rate, especially among the young, many researchers believe increases in life expectancy have ceased. (Do you know many obese people over 80 years old?) According to the Centers for Disease Control and Prevention, the percentage of children who are overweight has more than doubled since 1980.[9] In fact, according to a recent study, the factor that most increases a child's risk for being overweight is having obese parents.[10] Not only are we obese, but we are teaching our children to be obese and destining them to devastating obesity-related diseases.

New research findings linking obesity and poor lifestyle with various diseases are being published faster than I can read and summarized them. For each reference I have cited there are countless similar research articles. It is not necessary to find each and every study on the effects of poor lifestyle and being overweight to conclude that overwhelming evidence establishes that being fit, trim, making smart food choices, and getting adequate sleep offers huge benefits to health and longevity.

So to motivate you toward a healthier lifestyle, consider the benefits. The rewards of weight control and living healthfully include having a more vital, exciting life in a beautiful, stronger body. You can focus on making your dreams come true with the help of a strong, able body. The repercussions of obesity and an unhealthy lifestyle include a body that may hinder your ability to fulfill your dreams and an increased risk of developing debilitating diseases. While there are no guarantees of perfect health, being slim, fit, and strong can reduce disease risk and aid in the recovery from an illness. *If you truly want to lose weight and live the meaningful, exciting life you've dreamed of, make your decision today.*

---

[8] Archives of Internal Medicine v.163, p.1524, 2003

[9] Stanford magazine July/August 2004, p54

[10] Stanford Report, July 21, 2004

Chapter 2

The 3:00 PM Secret

Avoid continuous, permanent denial by adopting

a rhythm of 3:00 PM Days and Free Days

"Hi Isabelle! Heard you were back at work after your big trip to Tahiti. Nice tan!"

"Good to see you too, Josie. It was great."

"What's this I heard about rewarding yourself for sticking to some new fad diet? You know those never work," Josie said flicking her hair over her shoulder.

"Oh, it's not like that. Late last year I learned to adjust my eating style. Part of it is I don't eat much after 3:00 PM most days."

"That's crazy, Isabelle. I could never do that – I'd be ravenous! Besides, I like to reward myself at night with a treat for not eating as much during the day."

"You know, Josie, I was surprised that I'm really not hungry until breakfast. I also have time for myself at night rather than that old prepare, eat, clean up, get ready for bed routine."

"That reminds me," Josie interjected. "You know how I'm always trying to lose those twenty pounds? Well, I made a New Year's resolution to cut way back on my calories and to help me do that I skip breakfast. Problem is, by mid-morning I'm starving and feel tired, and I can't resist that pastry cart. Hey, here it comes now!"

Josie was off before Isabelle could explain the math – Isabelle was going 16 hours from her last meal until breakfast, with the last 8 hours asleep. Josie was trying to go 18 hours from dinner to lunch with the last several hours working at a low energy level – and failing without a Danish boost.

The 3:00 PM Secret:
A Rhythm of 3:00 PM Days and Free Days

There is a state of mind that often goes along with dieting and overeating, and there is a very different psychology that will enable long-term weight control. People embark on new "diets" anticipating they will be endlessly deprived. Eventually, they fall off the diet and overeat until the next attempt at endless dieting. There is a better, easier, and more natural way. By practicing *The 3:00 PM Secret*, you know you can eat a healthy, satisfying breakfast and lunch each day, and eat more freely every few days, yet still control your weight. As a result, you have no compulsion to overeat as if it may be your last satisfying meal.

A Digestion Detour

Let's step back, put on our lab coats, and consider what happens to the food we eat. When food is eaten, it is first digested and absorbed. Then it is used for energy and to build and maintain our bodies, and, if not immediately needed, stored as fat. Food that we eat early in the day can be burned off during the day's activities. If we eat late in the day or at night, and food is not burned through activity, much of it will be stored as fat during sleep.

During digestion the body transforms food into its basic components: carbohydrates, fats, proteins, vitamins, and minerals. The body absorbs these components, to build tissues and supply energy requirements. Digestion begins in the mouth, where food is partly broken down by chewing, and starches are further broken down by amylase enzymes. (*Starches* are a family of carbohydrates that consist of linked glucose molecules.) Food then proceeds through the esophagus to the stomach where it is further digested in strong gastric acid. After leaving the stomach, food enters the small intestine passing the bile duct opening in the duodenum, continues past the jejunum, and then the ilium (the final part of the small intestine). While in the small intestine, food continues to be broken down with the assistance of bile (which is produced in the liver and stored in the gall bladder). The food is also broken down by pancreatic enzymes and other digestive enzymes produced by the inner wall of the small intestine. In the small intestine, carbohydrates, fats, proteins, and vitamins are almost completely absorbed, and minerals are mostly absorbed. After leaving the small intestine, undigested fibers and waste products move to the large intestine where water and electrolytes (dissolved salts) are removed and where microbes produce a variety of vitamins, including biotin and vitamin K, and provide protection against infectious bacteria. Finally, solid waste is stored in the rectum until it is excreted via the anus.

Nutrient molecules absorbed through the small intestine are carried to the liver and other parts of the body in the bloodstream (or lymphatic system, then bloodstream). After carbohydrates, fats, and proteins are absorbed, they are used for energy, building body compounds, or they are stored. Carbohydrates are converted to glucose, which is used for energy. Proteins are broken down to amino acid components and used to replace body proteins. Protein can also be converted to glucose and used for energy if necessary. Fats are converted to fatty acids and glycerol (which can be converted to glucose) and also used for energy. Excess glucose is first stored as glycogen, but there is limited capacity of the glycogen-storing cells, so the surplus is stored as fat. Excess carbohydrates, proteins, and fats we eat are ultimately stored in fat cells. Glycogen, where glucose is first stored, can be readily converted back to glucose and used for energy.

The body's foremost concern is to meet energy requirements, which is accomplished by eating or by pulling from reserves, including glucose from stored glycogen and fatty acids from stored fat. If we eat early in the day while we are most active, we will use our food for energy throughout the day, and to support the body's functions (organ functions, brain and nervous system functions, and metabolic work of our cells). If we eat late in the day or in the evening when we are not active, less energy is required from our food and more of that food will go into storage as fat.

Does The Time Of Day When We Eat Matter?

If our goal is to lose weight and maintain a healthy weight, perhaps we can learn from people who succeed with the opposite goal: to gain and maintain a high weight. Sumo wrestlers want to gain and maintain a very high weight, because their livelihoods and reputations depend on it. So, how do Sumo wrestlers get so fat? They fast throughout the morning while they are exercising, eat a huge lunch, then nap several hours immediately after eating, which is crucial to their weight gain. After the afternoon nap, they may do further, though less rigorous, exercise, and then have their last large meal at night. Sumo wrestlers bulk up on Chankonabe, a boiled stew, which may include vegetables, fish, chicken, tofu, shrimp, beef, pork, noodles, and raw eggs, a large side of rice, and beer. If a wrestler is losing weight from strenuous training, he may add sugar-laden foods. Successful weight gain by Sumo wrestlers is credited to the large quantity of food eaten during their afternoon and evening meals in conjunction with the lack of activity after meals during digestion.[11] Skipping breakfast makes them hungrier so they can eat more. It is also believed overeating late in the day causes a drop in metabolism and encourages the body to store fat. After meals, sumo wrestlers sleep so most of the calories they eat will be deposited as fat.[12]

Interestingly, a study reported in the FDA Consumer Magazine in 2002 found that overweight people generally tend to skip breakfast,[13] thereby shifting their caloric intake later into the day and evening when they are less active. In fact, overweight people who are trying to diet tend to eat little or no breakfast, a light lunch, and consume most of their calories late in the day and at night. Conversely, this study found that people who successfully lose weight eat breakfast, thereby shifting calories earlier into the day. These successful weight losers also report they are physically active, monitor their weight frequently, and eat a lighter diet. People who successfully lose weight reject the pattern of skipping breakfast and eating more later in the day and adopt the pattern of eating breakfast, thereby shifting their food intake earlier into the day.

---

[11] The Wave Magazine Banzai Appetite; November 2002 issue of Saveur Magazine; http://www.pbs.org/independentlens/sumoeastandwest/sumo.html; http://oldeee.see.ed.ac.uk/~njt/Japanese/sumo.pdf

[12] http://www.discoverychannelasia.com/sumo/become_a_sumo_wrestler/index.shtml,Copyright © 2007 Discovery Comm. Inc

[13] January-February 2002, U.S. Food and Drug administration

Other research validating the benefits of eating earlier determined that people who eat more calories in the morning have been found to consume less calories overall for the day. A study of nearly 900 men and women reported in the Journal of Nutrition in January 2004 determined that the time of day people ate influenced the overall amount of food eaten that day.[14] It showed that the more food people ate in the morning, the fewer total calories they ate overall for that day. Conversely, when meals were eaten in the afternoon and evening, people ate more and had a greater overall daily intake of calories.

In a separate study reported in the American Journal of Clinical Nutrition in 1992, the role of breakfast in the treatment of obesity was evaluated.[15] Moderately obese women, some breakfast eaters and some breakfast skippers, were divided into two groups and assigned to a weight-loss program in which one group ate no breakfast and the other group ate breakfast. The researchers found that those who had to make the most substantial changes in eating habits to comply with the program achieved better results. They also found that eating breakfast helped reduce dietary fat and minimized impulsive snacking, and therefore may be an important part of a weight-reduction program.

It is interesting that making more substantial changes in one's eating program can lead to greater success. These studies are showing us that eating breakfast and shifting caloric intake earlier into the day helps people lose weight, eat fewer calories, and reduce dietary fat and impulsive snacking.

A further investigation pertaining to the detrimental effects of eating late in the day and evening was reported in Obesity Research in 2001 on the effects of night eating syndrome on weight loss.[16] In this study, participants were described as having night eating syndrome if they consumed more than 50% of total daily calories after 7 PM, skipped breakfast at least 4 days per week, and had difficulty falling asleep or staying asleep at least 4 days per week. Night eating syndrome was found to be associated with less weight loss in obese outpatients, along with depression, low self-esteem, and reduced daytime hunger. In this study, the night eaters lost less weight than the non-night eaters.

---

[14] Journal of Nutrition 134, p.104-111, January 2004, The American Society for Nutritional Sciences

[15] American Journal of Clinical Nutrition, v.55, p.645, 1992

[16] Obesity Research v.9, p.264, 2001; The North American Association for the Study of Obesity

In a study evaluating 714 patients with Type I and II diabetes, 9.7% of patients reported eating more than 25% of their daily food after their evening meal. Results revealed the night eaters had a significant association between night-eating symptoms and obesity. In fact, while "controlling for age, sex, race, and major depression, patients with night-eating behaviors, compared with patients without night-eating behaviors, were more likely to be obese." In addition, although the use of insulin was similar, adverse diabetes self-management and outcomes were evidenced. Night eaters also had more emotional problems.[17]

Night-eating syndrome was first described in 1955 by Stunkard and colleagues, and was characterized by morning anorexia, evening hyperphagia (excessive overeating), and insomnia.[18] It was more recently reported that although it does occur among non-obese people, night-eating syndrome appears to be more common among obese persons and increases in prevalence with increasing obesity.[19] In a study designed to assess the prevalence of night eating syndrome and its psychopathology in a psychiatric population, obese patients were found to be more likely than non-obese patients to have this syndrome.[20] In another study designed to evaluate hormones involved in energy balance, sleep, and stress in patients with night eating syndrome, it was noted that this syndrome is associated with obesity and depressed mood.[21] In addition, high rates of the night eating syndrome have been found in obese patients in bariatric (obesity) surgery clinics.[22]

Due to their job requirements, shift workers are active and eat at night. Researchers have noted that these people have an elevated risk of cardiovascular disease. It has also been found that, regardless of age or gender, an increasing duration of a person's shift work experience correlates with an increasing body mass index (see Appendix 2: Body Mass Index) and waist to hip ratio.[23] Because night work is becoming more prevalent, a group of researchers wanted to understand the impact of eating at different times of a 24 hour period, the effect on the body's metabolic responses, and whether dietary composition would affect these responses. The researchers pointed out the obvious – that "because the body's metabolic system is set for

---

[17] Diabetes Care v.29, p1800, 2006

[18] American Journal of Medicine v.19, No.1, p.78-86, 1955

[19] JAMA v.282, No.7, p657, 8/18/99

[20] Am J Psychiatry v.163, p156, January 2006

[21] The Journal of Clinical Endocrinology & Metabolism v.90, No.11, 6214, 2005

[22] Int J Eat Dis v.19, p.23, 1996/ Obesity Research v.12, p.1789, 2004

[23] Int J Obes Relat Metab Disord. v.23, No.9, p.973, Sept 1999

activity and meal intake during the day, and rest and fasting during the night, we anticipated a difference in metabolic response between day and night." The researchers noted that the makeup of our endocrine systems may be less suitable for food intake during the night and that the "nocturnal hormonal pattern" might be involved in the high incidence of obesity and cardiovascular diseases often seen in shift workers.[24]

Several studies have documented that many obese people eat more than half their daily calories at night. Some scientists think these people may have an abnormal internal clock mechanism in their brains which influences their eating times.[25]

A further argument for not eating at night is that it supports one of the primary lifestyle treatment guidelines for reducing gastroesophageal reflux disease (GERD), which is to avoid eating at night or within three to four hours before bedtime or lying down.[26]

These above mentioned studies indicate that when it comes to weight control, the time of day when we eat really *does* matter, and that it is particularly advantageous to eat earlier in the day when we tend to be more active, and to eat less in the evening when we are not as active and therefore likely to store the late-eaten calories as fat. Having a healthy, nutritious breakfast and lunch provides fuel to carry us through the day when we need energy and can burn what we eat. Unless we engage in energy-demanding activities at night, we should have eaten enough food to support our body's functions and sustain our energy as we wind down the day's activities.

You may ask whether eating about the same amount of food early versus late in the day really makes that much difference in how much a person weighs. This is difficult to measure since you cannot control all aspects of a person's behavior, including whether they deviate from some prescribed menu. There are secondary effects, however, from eating one's meals early in the day versus late in the day and at night. These effects include the physiological consequences of burning calories as we eat them early in the day when we are most active versus storing (in fat cells) most of what we eat at night when we are inactive.

---

[24] The American Society for Nutritional Sciences J. Nutr. 132:1892-1899, 2002

[25] Science news v.170, No.7, p.109, 8/12/06; (Nat. Acad. Sci. V.103, No.32, 12150-12155, August 8, 2006)

[26] American College of Gastroenterology, http://www.gastromd.com/education/gerd.html];
http://www.clevelandclinic.org/health/health-info/docs/1600/1697.asp?index=7042&src=news;
http://www.gicare.com/pated/ecdgs39.htm

There are also behavioral effects of eating most calories early rather than late. If we consume most of our food early and have a healthy satisfying breakfast and lunch, we are likely to have more energy and be more physically active during the day and burn more of what we have eaten. Alternatively, if we eat our meals late in the day and eat less food early in the day, we are likely to have less energy, be more lethargic, and burn fewer calories throughout the day as we drag ourselves around. In addition, if we have skipped breakfast, we may be more likely to eat some quick pick-me-up, unhealthy, high-calorie food such as a pastry. If we eat most of our food at the end of the day when we are already tired and winding down, we are likely to be less active and not burn the calories we would have burned if we had eaten them earlier in the day when we needed them for energy and activities. We may also be more likely to eat a greater number of calories overall when we shift our food consumption later into the afternoon and evening, as was pointed out in a study mentioned above. When we are up and busy with work, chores, and activities, we may be less likely to spend time overeating, whereas at night people tend to sit in front of the TV and unthinkingly consume more food at dinner and nighttime snacks than they would eat at lunch or breakfast.

You may find that satisfying your hunger in a healthy way early in the day and not eating at night is much easier than attempting to push away from the table during the dinner meal once you've gotten started eating – particularly since at night you may be tired and have limited self control. I believe eating healthy early in the day and not eating later in the day and at night is the secret to sustained weight control. You can satisfy your hunger early when you need food to sustain the activities of the day. Then, focus your evenings on the activities and pursuits that give your life meaning.

3:00 PM Days and Free Days

Imagine you are being forced to walk across a desert and it will take a long time – weeks, months, you're not sure. But you have to do it. The problem is water. You are not allowed to carry any water with you. Imagine there are two scenarios you could face regarding water and thirst on your journey across the desert.

Scenario 1: You are told there is water out there ... somewhere, and you are assured you will come across it ... sometime. You are allowed to drink water before you leave. Because you don't know when you will come across water, your natural inclination will be to drink so much it will make you feel sick. Then suppose you come across water sooner than you had expected. Again, your natural inclination will be to drink until you feel sick because you have the feeling it could be a very long time until you will come across water again.

Scenario 2: You are assured there is plenty of water every 2 miles during your entire trip. You will never be deprived of water; there will only be short delays until you walk 2 miles to the next water supply. Before you leave you are allowed to drink as much as you want. Are you going to drink until you feel sick? Of course not. There will be plenty of water again in 2 miles. When you get to each water supply, will you drink yourself sick? Probably not.

These two scenarios represent a mindset that also applies to food and dieting. When dieting, a person embarks on the diet anticipating he or she will be endlessly deprived. Sooner or later, the person falls off the diet and overeats until the next attempt at endless dieting and deprivation. Alternatively, by practicing *The 3:00 PM Secret*, you know you can eat a healthy, satisfying breakfast and lunch each day, and eat more freely every few days, yet still control your weight. There is no compulsion to overeat as if it may be your last satisfying meal.

Since the time of day we eat matters, and food eaten early in the day can be burned off during the day's activities, but food eaten late in the day or at night is not burned off through activity but rather stored as fat, then it makes sense to eat earlier and not eat at night. Yet, if we still want to regularly go out to dinner or have guests for dinner, then we must have certain nights when it is OK to eat dinner at the "normal" time. Therefore, we have *The 3:00 PM Secret* with a rhythm of *3:00 PM Days and Free Days*.

The 3:00 PM Secret involves not eating after 3:00 PM at least five days a week and having the remaining two days, if desired, as *Free days*. This results in a rhythm of *3:00 PM days* and *Free days*. *The 3:00 PM Secret* will balance the amount of food you consume over a several day period, and allow you to get the average number of calories each day that is appropriate for the weight you desire to support. *The 3:00 PM Secret* advocates intermittent periods of several days of highly-nutritious light eating when you only eat early during the day (up to 3:00 PM), followed by one or two days of free but healthy eating when you can eat more freely later in the day, then back to *3:00 PM days*, then *Free days*, and so on. It will take a few months to get into a comfortable rhythm and some time to fine-tune how much you eat and the timing and number of *3:00 PM days* and *Free days*. Once you are comfortable with a rhythm that works for you, you will never have to face the prospect of continuous, daily, permanent self-denial to achieve and maintain your desired body. *This method works because virtually everyone can exercise self-control over their eating for a few days if they are rewarded with a day or two of not having to be so controlled. It is also easy to exercise self-control by not eating a meal at night if you can look forward to a satisfying and healthy breakfast.*

If you are concerned about not eating between 3:00 PM and the next morning, a period of 15 or 16 hours, consider that many people skip breakfast and eat their first meal at noon. These breakfast skippers go without food from sometime between 6:00 PM and 9:00 PM at night until 12:00 PM the next day, which is *the same or more hours without food as The 3:00 PM Secret suggests,* just at the wrong times. In addition, people on a more traditional schedule eat dinner at 5:00 PM and don't eat after 6:00 PM, so there is only a three-hour difference between not eating after 3:00 PM and not eating after 6:00 PM. Also, *The 3:00 PM Secret* does allow vegetable juice, milk/soymilk, a piece of fruit, etc., in the evening, and for those going out at night, it recommends having a piece of fruit or milk/soymilk, etc. *The 3:00 PM Secret* does not require any extended fasting.

Note that if you do not work a standard 8:00 AM to 5:00 PM day job and sleep at night, but rather work at night and sleep during the day, then you can practice *The 3:00 PM Secret* by eating breakfast upon awakening, eating a nutritious lunch and snack if needed, and then refrain from eating within six hours of going to bed.

You do not need to abruptly start *The 3:00 PM Secret*, but can begin getting used to the *3:00 PM days* by slowly moving up your last meal of the day. Begin by not eating after 5:00 PM five days a week for one or two weeks, then stop eating by 4:30 PM for one or two weeks, then 4:00 PM for one or two weeks, then 3:30 PM, and then 3:00 PM (or earlier).

Note: It is important that you discuss this new eating style with your doctor (especially if you have or are prone to diabetes) and verify that he or she confirms that not eating between 3:00 PM and 6:00 AM the next morning 5 days a week is acceptable for you. If your doctor believes you should eat after 3:00 PM, you can make it a light meal. In addition, on any *3:00 PM day* you can have a glass of milk/soymilk, a cup of clear soup, a piece of fruit, or other light, nutritious snack if needed in the evening.

Examples of The 3:00 PM Secret rhythm: By having *3:00 PM days*, when you consume less food and calories, combined with *Free days*, when you consume more food and calories, you will average out the total calories consumed over a period of a week. The following are examples of how someone may average the amount of food consumed on *3:00 PM days* and *Free days*. In these examples, I am specifying *calories* to clarify the concept of averaging what you consume. I am not, however, recommending counting calories as a daily practice. Most people can tell if they are eating lightly or eating heavily. Over time you will be able to adjust how much you are eating on *3:00 PM days* and *Free days* to bring yourself to the weight you desire. People are often surprised how little food their bodies require, provided it is nutritious.

As a reference, the following are general recommended guidelines for numbers of calories to consume each day as suggested on the www.metlife.com web page:

• Sedentary women and older adults: 1,600 calories/day.

• Children, teenage girls, active women, sedentary men: 2,200 calories/day.

• Teenage boys, active men, very active women: 2,800 calories/day.

Individuals will vary in the number of calories they can handle based on the muscle content of their body, how active they are, and other individual factors. Three possible examples of using the *3:00 PM days* and *Free days* rhythm to average the amount of food you consume in a week are listed below.

> ***Example 1***: You are an active woman, a sedentary man, or a teenage girl and your optimum caloric intake is approximately 2200 calories/day. To consume an average of 2200 calories/day over a week you can choose:
>
> • Five *3:00 PM days* per week, (Monday through Friday), and eat 1700 calories/day.
>
> • Two *Free days* per week, (Saturday and Sunday), and eat 3450 calories/day.

Example 2: You are a sedentary woman or older adult and your optimum calories are 1600 calories/day. To consume an average of 1600 calories/day over a week you can choose:

- Five *3:00 PM days* per week, (Monday through Friday), and
  eat 1200 calories/day.

- Two *Free days* per week, (Saturday and Sunday), and
  eat 2600 calories/day.

Example 3: You are a very active woman, an active man, or a teenage boy and your optimum caloric intake is approximately 2800 calories/day. To consume an average of 2793 calories/day over a week you can choose:

- Four *3:00 PM days* per week, (Monday through Thursday), and
  eat 2000 calories/day.

- Three *Free days* per week, (Friday through Sunday), and
  eat 3850 calories/day.

Your 3:00 PM days and *Free days can be grouped together or interspersed.* Also, holidays marked by special meals such as Thanksgiving really ought to be scheduled as *Free Days*! The *Free days* may be together, such as Friday and Saturday or Saturday and Sunday as *Free days* with the remaining days as *3:00 PM days*. Alternatively, *Free days* may also be separated, such as Wednesday and Saturday as *Free days* and Monday, Tuesday, Thursday, Friday, and Sunday as *3:00 PM days*. You can vary the timing of *3:00 PM days* and *Free days* from week to week. As you get into a rhythm of eating more some days and less other days, you will easily begin to judge how it is affecting your weight and whether you want to cut back on what you are eating on *3:00 PM days,* or change the ratio of *3:00 PM days* and *Free days,* or do some combination of the two. The actual number of days that are your *3:00 PM days* and the number of days that are your *Free days* will depend on your height, bone structure, muscle mass, metabolism, level of exercise, and desired weight, as well as the amount of food you consume. Unless you are a teenage boy, an active man, or a very active woman, I recommend that you choose at least five *3:00 PM days* each week.

You can also use this strategy in combination with a particular diet that you choose, such as a diet prescribed by your doctor, a low-carbohydrate diet, or a vegetarian diet. In addition, on *3:00 PM days* you may decide to eat two larger meals or several smaller meals up to 3:00 PM. Give yourself several months to get completely comfortable with this new eating style and to work out what amounts of foods to eat on *3:00 PM days* and on *Free days*. You will be able to obtain and maintain your desired weight by optimizing how much you eat on *3:00 PM days* and *Free days*, limiting the number of *Free days*, eating highly nutritious foods, consistently doing the ten-minute workout, and getting adequate sleep. Finally, the use of *Free days* serves two purposes: the first is for the psychological benefit of making it easier to maintain the *3:00 PM days*, and the second is to allow social dinner engagements. Some people will find no need for the psychological reward system, and will enjoy the advantages of making nearly all days *3:00 PM days*, with a few exceptions such as evenings when they have a social dinner engagement. This is the pattern that works best for me. I prefer to eat early in the day and not eat at night unless I have a social engagement. When I do eat at night, I keep it light or I don't sleep well. I can't imagine going back to a lifestyle of eating a main meal at night. I love having my nights free from the dinner preparation, eating, and cleanup routine.

If you are thinking that it seems unfathomable not to eat after 3:00 PM, consider the alternative. There are successfully trim people who manage a lifetime of continual, consistent, permanent, daily self-denial from eating as much as they want of their favorite foods. While this approach does work for some people, most of us find this strategy of weight control too depressing to seriously contemplate. It *is* possible, however, to practice an easy, relatively painless eating strategy that will give you a life-long method for total control over your body without constant denial. The *rhythm* of *3:00 PM days* and *Free days* along with proper nutrition, a short daily physical workout, and adequate sleep offers an easy, painless way to control your weight and look your best. You can go out to dinner once or twice a week if you feel like it, or have weekend company and enjoy yourself.

Do you think you can be happy to have five *3:00 PM* days a week if you can eat more freely two days a week and still have the body you desire? It is easy to eat less on *3:00 PM days* when you can eat more freely on *Free days* and you are living in, or noticeably approaching, your ideal body. It is also easy to skip dinner when you can enjoy an activity you thought you didn't have time for, sleep well, and look forward to getting up to a healthy, satisfying breakfast. After several months, you will find having *3:00 PM days* and *Free days* very easy to maintain, and may eventually prefer *3:00 PM days*. Expect it to take a few months to become comfortable with this eating style. Then you will realize you have found an easy method to achieve permanent weight control without endlessly having to restrain yourself from eating your favorite foods. It also is likely that you will actually feel better and sleep better on *3:00 PM days* without having your stomach so full of food, and may choose to limit eating at night to social events and special dinners. In fact, once you become used to eating early and not stuffing yourself at night, you will find that you not only sleep better but also have more free time because you will open up your evenings to do more enjoyable activities than being a slave to a dinner planning, production, consumption, and cleanup routine.

If you have a mate or children who are slim, active, and either need or insist on evening meals, you still can prepare a healthy dinner for them and save your portion in the refrigerator and enjoy it the next day for lunch. If your spouse is also overweight, why not invite him or her to join you in your new pattern of eating. If you have overweight children or teenagers, you may assist them in shifting their food intake earlier in the day, and perhaps serve a fruit salad or other light healthy snack for dinner rather than a heavy meal. Remember, they are forming habits for a lifetime.

Eating in a *rhythm* of having *3:00 PM days* and *Free days* will allow you to break the pattern of habit-eating (eating from habit rather than true hunger) as well as end the psychology of permanent self-denial, which can lead to binge eating. There is never a need to overeat because you can eat more freely every few days for the rest of your life and still feel satisfied, and you can have a satisfying, healthy breakfast every day. *3:00 PM days* should be used to focus on nutritious eating and supplying basic energy requirements, and *Free days* can be used to consume nutritious foods, but also provide pleasure eating in order to eliminate the feeling of endless deprivation. The rhythm or pattern of *3:00 PM days* and *Free days* can accomplish several important benefits:

1. Allows an optimal average daily food intake to maintain your desired body size.

2. Provides a psychologically-appealing method of short-term periods of self-control interspersed with days of eating more freely, avoiding feelings of endless, daily deprivation.

3. Provides an easy way to eat less overall since it takes less self control to not eat a meal at night than it does to push away from the dinner table once you've started eating.

4. Gives you the food energy early in the day when you need it and will burn the calories you eat, rather than if you eat at night when you are not as active and are less likely to burn the food you eat for energy.

5. Breaks the destructive habit of continual stuffing or habit eating. Once you get used to not constantly overeating on your *3:00 PM days*, you will eventually break the pattern of habit eating.

6. Ends the unfavorable practice of *night eating,* when unneeded calories are not burned for energy but stored as fat.

7. Supports one of the primary lifestyle treatment guidelines for reducing gastroesophageal reflux disease (GERD), which is to avoid eating at night or within three to four hours of bedtime or lying down.[27]

8. Nullifies one of the psychological reasons that can initiate a pattern of binge eating, which is to overeat for several days as a prelude to a *diet.* Dieters let themselves overeat with the promise that they will then exercise endless self-control and denial. Unfortunately, they then find the diet too endlessly restrictive and after some period of self-restraint they have had enough, and return to their old routine of constant overeating. At some time in the future they get motivated again to lose weight and once again have their "last" big binge before their "last" big diet, which eventually fails because once again they can't face a future of never-ending self-restraint and denial. This turns into a vicious, frustrating, and unnecessary cycle of bingeing and dieting.

Instead of attempting endless self-control and denial to control weight, it seems much more appealing to practice limited self-restraint for a few days if you know you can eat more freely for a couple of days. If you practice a *rhythm* of *3:00 PM days* and *Free days*, there is no compulsion for a "last binge" because for the rest of your life you can eat more freely a couple of

---

[27] http://www.gastromd.com/education/gerd.html;
http://www.clevelandclinic.org/health/health-info/docs/1600/1697.asp?index=7042&src=news;
http://www.gicare.com/pated/ecdgs39.htm

days each week. Also, on *3:00 PM days,* you can exercise a few hours of self-control and refrain from eating dinner knowing you can wake up to a healthy breakfast. Yes, there are various other reasons people binge. However, when a person gets into this type of eating pattern and sticks to it, it may be possible to develop the ability to achieve short periods of self-control. With this approach, there is no endless denial, so there is no need to ever overeat. This type of eating rhythm also gives the body periods of rest from being filled with heavy foods.

The rhythm of *3:00 PM days* and *Free days* provided by *The 3:00 PM Secret* is not so different from what our friends in the animal kingdom do naturally. Eating more heavily on some days and lightly on other days is a natural rhythm for many wild animals as well as many people who may not have been trained or forced to eat the traditional three meals every single day, three hundred sixty-five days a year. Wild animals generally do not eat three meals a day, each and every day. Cats, such as the bobcat, frequently fast for some time when food is not available, then eat heavily when it is available. Other wild animals will eat heavily for a day or two, then eat lightly until they get hungry at which time they go in search of another meal. Sometimes human infants and young children have a natural hunger cycle in which they are not particularly hungry for a few days and then eat a lot when they eventually get hungry. As they grow up, however, they are trained to conform to the three-meals-per-day, three hundred sixty-five days per year cultural norm. Unfortunately, obesity has also become a cultural norm.

Most "diets" provide a program to lose weight and then a second program for "maintenance". Initially, people are often able to lose weight, but they gain it back once they go off the diet and into "maintenance" mode letting their guard down. There is no such thing as "maintenance" if it is interpreted as "go back to normal". If you want to maintain a new lower weight, you will not be able to go back to the lifestyle that made you heavy in the first place. What you did to get slim, you must continue to do, to some degree, in order to maintain your desired weight. That means continuing some form of *3:00 PM days* and *Free days indefinitely*. I am convinced that once you get used to *3:00 PM days*, you will never want to give them up as a normal eating pattern, as the benefits of not eating at night are remarkably positive.

Self-Control On 3:00 PM Days

Use 3:00 PM days to take your focus off food and begin to think about, investigate, and pursue what fascinates you and would bring purpose, adventure, and meaning into your life.

The first rule of self-control: The easiest place to exercise self-control over what you eat is at your front door. If you don't want to eat something on a *3:00 PM day*, keep it out of your house. If one of your favorite foods is in your house and you are having a weak moment, it will be extremely difficult not to eat it. If you have not been able to manage your weight, then you know that consistently exercising self-control is a problem. It is not reasonable to expect yourself all of a sudden to be able to conjure up unwavering control on your *3:00 PM days*, just because you will have *Free days*. So make it easier on yourself by not having to resist food that is too accessible. Eat selected favorite foods on your *Free days*, but keep them out of your house on your *3:00 PM days*. Even though you manage to control your own behavior with respect to keeping favorite foods out of your house on *3:00 PM days*, you can rest assured that well-meaning family and friends will show up at the door with harmful treats. So be prepared to ask them to leave their treats in their car and take them back home when they leave.

The second rule of self-control: Remove trigger foods. Many of your favorite foods may be what are sometimes referred to as "trigger foods". Trigger foods are foods that you find yourself continually overeating; they are the ones that you can't seem to eat in reasonable portions. Please keep trigger foods out of your house at least on *3:00 PM days*. If one of your trigger foods happens to be a favorite food of one of your family members and he (or she) thinks he just has to keep it on hand, it may be helpful to offer to do one of his chores if he agrees not to keep certain foods in the house, especially on your *3:00 PM days*. For example, offer to wash his car once a week or take over a yard work chore (or hire someone else to do it) if he will keep your trigger food out of the house. Make his sacrifice worthwhile so you can do everything possible to avoid having your efforts sabotaged.

The third rule of self-control: Manage the need to feed others at night. A potential obstacle to not eating at night is the need to feed others. If you have children and a mate who are slim, active, and either need or insist on evening meals, you can still prepare a healthy dinner for them and save your portion in the refrigerator overnight to enjoy the next day for lunch. As mentioned above, if they are overweight, you can help them shift their food intake earlier in the day as well and invite them to join you on *3:00 PM days*.

The fourth rule of self-control: Have something soothing to drink to take the edge off nighttime hunger. If you are finding it difficult to not eat at night on *3:00 PM days*, and you feel as if you need something in your stomach, have a cup of clear soup or warm milk, a cup of soymilk/milk, a cup of tea with milk, a glass of juice, a piece of fruit, or something similar.

The fifth rule of self-control: Go grocery shopping on *Free days* and purchase only enough of your Free-day foods for the immediate *Free day(s)* plus the foods you plan to have in your house to eat on your *3:00 PM days*. *3:00 PM-d*ay foods should be highly nutritious foods that you do not have a tendency to overeat. In addition, avoid grocery shopping on an empty stomach so you don't overbuy *Free-day* foods. If you end up having some of your Free-day foods left over that you don't want to eat on *3:00 PM days*, take them to someone else's house to hold for you for a few days or give them to a food bank. Don't sabotage yourself by buying large quantities of your favorite foods that you eat on *Free days* or you will end up eating those foods against your will on your *3:00 PM days*. It may seem as if you are saving money by purchasing food in bulk, but you're not saving money on foods that you end up overeating. For example, if you want some peanuts on your *Free days* and a small bag costs $1 and a bag four-times larger costs only $2, then it may seem prudent to buy the larger 'money-saving' bag. But in reality, if you end up eating the entire bag whether it is the small bag or the large bag, and you buy the large bag, then, at the end of the day, you have wasted an extra dollar on peanuts and you have overeaten.

The sixth rule of self-control: Turn off your television. There is a large and undeniable correlation between television watching and obesity. In a six year study of 50,000 women as part of the Nurse's Health Study, when exercise, smoking, diet, and age were controlled, it was found that each 2-hour increase in daily television watching was associated with a 23% increase in obesity and a 7% increase in diabetes risk.[28] If you must waste time, find a better way than watching television!

The seventh rule of self-control: One of the best ways to enhance self-control on your *3:00 PM days* is to use your *3:00 PM days* to transfer the energy you normally expend on food planning, preparation, and cleanup to investigating

---

[28] Science v. 300, No. 5618, p421, 4/18/03

how you can transform your life and move toward a future that will give your life purpose and adventure. Instead of sitting on the couch watching food-filled commercials, go to a bookstore or library, or search the internet, and look through articles, magazines and books on the subjects that you may truly find fascinating and could lead to a more meaningful and exciting future. If you already have or discover interests or hobbies that can lead to a more adventurous life, begin investigating or participating in them during your evenings.

The other side of calories: If you are eternally frustrated that your body's overall caloric needs are much less than what you wish you could consume without gaining weight, here are a few points to keep in mind that may make you feel better. Eating fewer but more nutritious calories as a regular practice has been shown to increase lifespan! In addition, requiring fewer calories is also a survival benefit. Requiring fewer calories to sustain our bodies is a survival benefit because we don't have to obtain a large amount of food every day just to stay alive. Many people may wish they could consume 3 to 5 thousand calories per day and not gain weight, but consider our ability to survive if our bodies actually required large numbers of calories to maintain a healthy weight and prevent starvation! Remember, in many parts of the world, people struggle to obtain the minimum amount of nutrition required for a healthy body. If all humans actually required 3, 4, or 5 thousand calories every day to survive, world starvation would be an epidemic, and the cost of producing all that food would be astronomical! So when you get frustrated that you seem to gain or maintain an undesirable weight on what seems like not very many calories, think about how expensive and burdensome it would be if you and your loved ones withered away and starved to death on anything less than 4 or 5 thousand calories a day. (I hope this helps.)

Chapter 3

Ten Tips for Good Nutrition

and Foods to Emphasize

"Oh, excuse me," Isabelle said as she backed into a library table knocking a stack of biology books to the floor.

"No problem, I was getting tired of studying anyway. Ah, hi, my name is Trevor."

Isabelle didn't notice Trevor extending his hand to shake hers as she reached down to pick up the books. "Wow, look at this, a book on the diets of wild animals. That's interesting. I read that many wild animals eat a lot and then don't eat much for a few days." Nice eyes, Isabelle thought at she looked up.

"Yes, that's true, particularly for carnivores and wild cats. But what's really fascinating is that wild animals possess an amazing ability to select a diet that meets their nutritional requirements, and yet they avoid eating significant amounts of poisonous or toxic substances."

"Really?"

"Yes, and somehow they can recognize a food's nutritional value, which is not necessarily related to the food's taste or smell." Trevor was staring back at Isabelle.

"Do you think we possess this ability instinctively as well?" Isabelle raised her eyebrow.

"Now that's a thought-provoking question." Trevor rubbed his chin.

"You sound very scientific. Are you a veterinarian?" Isabelle asked.

"A veterinarian and a student. I am actually going back to school for a PhD in biology. I'm really more interested in studying animals in the wild, in their natural habitats. What about you? What brings you out to the library on a Friday night?"

"I am exploring what may interest me. Its funny, until I read this book on weight control, I never really thought about what I truly want to do with my life. I just sort of blindly went forward, got a boring degree, and an even more boring job. Now I'm giving myself the chance to find something that really interests me. I've always liked geology"

"I can relate to that...What did you say your name was?" Trevor smiled back at Isabelle.

Do we instinctively possess the ability to know whether a food is nutritious or toxic? It *is* a thought-provoking question, particularly because left to our appetites, we humans often overeat non-nutritious, unhealthy foods while under-eating nutritious, healthy foods. This often leads to obese yet somewhat malnourished bodies.

All animals, including humans, must balance their nutrient intake with their body's metabolic demands by regulating what and when they eat. If we provide our bodies with optimum nutrition, we can positively affect our health and lifespan. People in some cultures have better health and longer life spans than others. It is believed that dietary habits play a large role in keeping them healthy and living longer.

DIET AND CULTURE: Three types of diets are widely believed to be associated with good health and longevity. These are the traditional Japanese, Chinese, and Mediterranean diets.[29]   Life expectancy in Japan is the highest in the world, with low death rates from heart disease.[30]   The Japanese diet is high in omega-3 ("good") fat-containing fish, mineral rich seaweeds, rice, vegetables, miso (fermented soybean paste), and tofu, while it is low in saturated ("bad") fat-containing red meat and dairy. On Okinawa the death rates caused by strokes, cancer, and heart disease are even lower than in other parts of Japan. Okinawans consume three-times more vegetables, twice as much fish, only 20% of the salt, and only 25% of the sugar of other Japanese.

The traditional Chinese diet is rich in vegetables, rice, tofu, and green tea, as well as garlic, onions, and ginger. The traditional Chinese diet has more fruits, vegetables, fish, and plant proteins, and less dairy products, meat, and sugar than the western diet.[31]

The traditional Mediterranean diet is rich in olive oil (monounsaturated fats), vegetables, fish, legumes, fruits, nuts, and cereals, with a moderate intake of alcohol, mostly in the form of wine at meals. It is low in saturated fats, with a low-to-moderate intake of dairy products (mostly yogurt or cheese), and a low intake of meat and poultry. The traditional Mediterranean diet supplies as much as 40% of total daily calories from fat (mostly monounsaturated and polyunsaturated), yet the associated incidence of cardiovascular diseases is significantly decreased.[32]   The Mediterranean diet is associated with positive benefits in cardiovascular disease, lipoprotein profile, blood pressure, inflammation, glucose metabolism, antithrombotic profile, endothelial function, antioxidant properties, age-related cognitive decline, Alzheimer's disease, and healthier aging and increased longevity.[33] Together with regular physical activity and not smoking, it has been suggested that over 80% of coronary heart disease, 70% of stroke, and 90% of Type II diabetes can be avoided by healthy food choices that are consistent with the traditional Mediterranean diet.[34]

---

[29]   N. Engl. J. Med. v.344, p940, Mar 2001

[30]   Professor Yasuo Kagawa, Jichi Medical School, Tochigi-Ken, Japan

[31]   http://www.eurekalert.org/pub_releases/1999-11/AHA-TCdh-091199.php,
       http://www.birmingham.gov.uk/GenerateContent?CONTENT_ITEM_ID=909&CONTENT_ITEM_TYPE=0&MENU_ID=10084&EXPAND=10071

[32]   http://www.hsph.harvard.edu/press/releases/press06252003.html

[33]   Eur J Clin Invest v.35, No.7, p421, Jul 2005

[34]   Public Health Nutr. v.9, No.1A, p.105, Feb 2006

What common features do we find in these apparently healthier diets? An emphasis on vegetables, unsaturated fats in the form of fish and olive oil, fruits, soy (tofu), and whole grains, as well as a de-emphasis on sugar, processed foods, meat and dairy. There are also a few bonus foods, such as mineral rich seaweeds, garlic, ginger, wine, and green tea.

Another country with an enviable statistic is India. The rates of Alzheimer's disease are much lower among the elderly in India than in the West, which has prompted interest in determining the cause of their particularly low incidence of the disease. The reduction in Alzheimer's disease in India may very likely be explained by the generous use of the Indian spice turmeric. The active compound, curcumin, derived from the curry spice *turmeric*, has an extensive history as a food additive and herbal medicine in India. It is a potent antioxidant, and may play a role in slowing down the progression of Alzheimer's disease. Studies on curcumin (in turmeric) suggest that it shows promise for the prevention of Alzheimer's disease[35] and may play a role in slowing down the progression of the disease.[36] A Singapore study suggests curcumin may counter cognitive decline.[37] Other research suggests that curcumin, present in turmeric, may also be an effective protective agent against cataract formation,[38] and may have anti-inflammatory, anti-cancer, and anti-tumor benefits.[39] More recent studies have also focused on its potential anti-cancer properties.[40]

It is also worth mentioning some recent statistics on *vegetarian* diets. A recent review of vegetarians and non-vegetarians revealed that vegetarians tend to weigh less than non-vegetarians and have a lower incidence of certain diseases associated with overweight and obese individuals, such as heart disease, high blood pressure, certain cancers, and diabetes,[41] particularly Type II diabetes.[42] While rates of obesity in the general population are rising dramatically, rates of obesity in vegetarians range from 0 to 6 percent. In fact, the authors of the review found that the body weight of both male and female vegetarians is, on average, 3 to 20 percent lower than that of meat-eaters. In this review the authors compiled data from 87 previous studies and

[35] The Journal of Neuroscience v.21, No.21, p.8370, 11/1/01

[36] BBC NEWS, 11/21/01 http://news.bbc.co.uk/2/hi/health/1668932.stm

[37] American Journal of Epidemiology Nov. 1 2006/ Science News v.170, No.20, p.316, 11/11/06

[38] American Journal of Clinical Nutrition v.64, 761, 1996

[39] Carcinogenesis, v.20, No.5, p.911, May 1999; Carcinogenesis v.14, p.493, 1993 by Oxford University Press; American Journal of Clinical Nutrition v.70, No.3, p.491, September 1999

[40] Science News, v.166, No.15, p.238, 10/9/04

[41] Nutrition Reviews v.64, No.4, p.175, April 2006

[42] Am J Clin Nutr. v.78, No.3 Suppl, p.610, Sept 2003

found that a vegetarian diet is highly effective for weight loss, which occurs at a rate of approximately 1 pound per week, and that the weight-loss effect does not depend on exercise or calorie-counting. Emphasizing plant foods in your diet is healthy as a general practice. It has been shown that a high consumption of plant-based foods such as fruits and vegetables, nuts, and whole grains is associated with a significantly lower risk of coronary artery disease and stroke.[43]

This book does not focus on any particular diet, but rather on achieving and sustaining weight-control through optimal nutrition, the ten-minute workout, healthy sleep, and the use of *3:00 PM days* in a psychologically-pleasing *3:00 PM day* and *Free day* rhythm that can be followed for life. Recipes are not included in this book, but rather types of foods to emphasize are suggested, as well as the types of foods to avoid or limit. There are many excellent books available that contain healthy and interesting recipes.

You may prefer to eat a diet based on certain nutritional principles, including the Japanese, traditional Chinese, and Mediterranean diets, diets rich in olive oil and fish, diets emphasizing low-carbohydrate foods, diets emphasizing a balance of protein, fat, and carbohydrates, or diets that are more vegetarian. Determine what works for you. In any diet you follow, however, try to incorporate the information in the *Ten Tips For Good Nutrition* and *What Foods to Emphasize on 3:00 PM Days and Free Days* listed below. If you are on an extreme high-carbohydrate, low-fat, low-protein diet, you should limit the amount of sugar and processed carbohydrates you are consuming, and be careful that you are getting sufficient amounts of essential amino acids from proteins as well as the essential fatty acids and monounsaturated fatty acids from beneficial fats. Protein and fat are essential to healthy maintenance of our bodies. The typical American diet is way too high in sugar, which contributes to obesity, insulin resistance, diabetes, fatigue, and other health problems and diseases.

If your goal is to control your weight, remember that a key ingredient of any successful weight control plan is eating highly nutritious foods. If you are not providing yourself with optimal nutrition, you won't feel good, and will be tempted to overeat in order to boost your energy. If you weaken your body through inadequate nutrition, you will crave unnecessary calories as your body tries to get the nutrients it needs. Nutrition is an important key to weight control success! Eating good and healthful foods that are low in

---

sugar, processed carbohydrates, and unhealthy fats will make you feel better and help you control your temptation to overeat. If you eat junk food and fill up with sugar, you will feel drained and scattered, and may even cause yourself to be both malnourished and overweight. *3:00 PM days* should not consist of 4 candy bars and *Free days* 12 candy bars. It is critical to find foods you really like, but that also supply optimal nutrition. You may need to acquire new tastes, but if you limit unhealthy foods, you will eventually stop missing them.

Everything you eat or drink will go into your body and affect it in either a positive or negative way. Eating nutritious, high-quality foods will enhance your body and make you feel better, whereas eating unhealthy foods and empty calories will negatively affect your body over the long-term. It is important to eat wholesome, nutritious foods on both *3:00 PM days* and *Free days*. Good nutrition, exercise, and mental stimulation will enhance the quality of your life well into old age and keep your body younger longer. Who wants to become feeble and decrepit unnecessarily? It is definitely preferable to extend a vital and healthy life.

The Ten Tips For Good Nutrition

Avoid glutens + oils.
Eat eggs.
DARL 2016

In the confusing maze of dietary do's and don'ts, where fads come and go, it is essential to rely on information that is based on solid research studies and is consistent with the physiological makeup of our bodies. The following are general guidelines for maximizing nutrition.

1. Eat *vegetables* daily such as spinach, broccoli, chard, kale, purple cabbage, cauliflower, onions, garlic, parsley, red and green peppers, and other highly colored vegetables. If you don't eat vegetables daily, then drink fresh vegetable juices.

2. Eat *fruit* daily such as grapefruit, blueberries, strawberries, apricots, tangerines, apples, lemons, oranges, figs, raspberries, peaches, plums, cantaloupe, cherries, pears, grapes, and kiwis. If you don't eat fruit daily, then drink fresh low-sugar fruit juices.

3. Regularly consume *omega-3* and *omega-6 essential fatty acids* as well as *mono-unsaturated fatty acids*. The *omega-3* fatty acids should be emphasized. The most concentrated sources of *omega-3* fatty acids

include fatty and cold-water fish such as salmon and tuna, flaxseed oil, fish oil supplements, and omega-3 fatty acid supplements. Additional sources of omega-3 fatty acids include pumpkin seeds, walnuts, flaxseeds, and canola oil. High quality sources of omega-6 can be found in health-food stores and include evening primrose oil, borage oil, black currant seed oil, and gooseberry oils. More common healthy sources of *omega-6* fatty acids include raw nuts and seeds, legumes, leafy green vegetables, and grains. Vegetable oils, such as corn, safflower, sunflower, soybean, cottonseed, and sesame also contain omega-6 fatty acids, however these oils are generally processed and hydrogenated and should be limited because they contain harmful transfats. It is recommended that we consume a balance of omega-6 and omega-3 rich foods. Because omega-6 rich foods are far more prevalent, we need to pay attention to getting enough omega-3 rich foods. The *monounsaturated fatty acids* also have tremendous health benefits and should be included in your diet. Good sources of monounsaturated fatty acids include olive oil, canola oil, avocados, and nuts.

4. Consume sufficient *protein*, which can be obtained from various foods including fish and seafood such as salmon and tuna, nuts, seeds, nut and seed butters, tofu, soybeans, tempeh, beans, legumes, wheat germ, sprouted beans and grains, organic yogurt, and moderate amounts of animal protein such as organic cottage cheese and eggs.

5. Choose *whole-food complex carbohydrates* such as black, pinto, navy, and lima beans, peas, legumes, lentils, brown rice, wild rice, oats, unprocessed whole grains including buckwheat, millet, amaranth, quinoa, barley, rye, bulgur, whole-grain pumpernickel, wheat kernels, wheat grain, wheat germ, cracked wheat, cracked wheat bread, barley grain, and sprouts from vegetables, sunflowers, beans, and grains.

6. Talk to your doctor about taking multivitamin and mineral supplements, and if you are primarily vegetarian also ask about taking additional vitamin-B12 and zinc supplements.

7. Drink plenty of water (8 glasses a day are usually recommended). Avoid soft drinks, sugary drinks, and low calorie drinks with unhealthy artificial sweeteners.

8. Limit sugars, processed carbohydrates, and high-glycemic index carbohydrates such as sugar, white flour, muffins, pastries, sugary commercial breakfast cereals, honey, white breads and bagels, most crackers, white rice, cookies, chips, and jams.

9. Avoid or limit foods containing *transfats* including margarine, fried foods, vegetable shortening, hydrogenated vegetable oils, commercial pastries and baked food products containing hydrogenated oils (such as many breads, biscuits, cakes, cookies, crackers, doughnuts, muffins, pies and rolls), and most prepared snacks, mixes, and convenience foods. You may need to slowly wean yourself off these types of foods.

10. Avoid raw meats and raw eggs. Also, avoid raw fish if you have an impaired health defense system.[44]

It is helpful to focus on eating specific types of nutritious foods, such as those mentioned in tips 1 though 5 above, as well as the foods listed in the following section: *What Foods to Emphasize on 3:00 PM Days and Free Days*. Concentrating on eating several types of good foods each day will leave less time and energy for thinking about and eating junk foods. Focus on getting a healthy dose of vitamins, minerals, antioxidants, essential fatty acids, protein, and other nutrients. The above "Ten Tips" are discussed in detail in this chapter in the section *What Foods to Emphasize on 3:00 PM Days and Free Days*, and also in *Appendix 1: Essential Nutrients and Where to Find Them* in the sections *Vegetables, Fruits and Plant-Based Foods*; *Fats*; *Protein*; and *Sugars and Carbohydrates*.

What Foods to Emphasize on 3:00 PM Days and Free Days

On both *3:00 PM days* and *Free days*, it is beneficial to observe the suggestions given in *The Ten Tips For Good Nutrition* section above. Focus on eating nutritious foods every day. These foods should include vegetables, fruits, protein such as fish and soy, healthy fats such as flaxseed oil, fish oil, and olive oil, and whole foods such as nuts, legumes, and whole grains. Following is a list of nourishing foods from the vegetables, fruits, fats, protein, and carbohydrates groups that can be used to make healthy choices

---

[44] www.cfsan.fda.gov/~ear/FLRECSAF.htm

in your daily diet. It is not a complete listing of what is healthy and nutritious, but rather good examples of foods and types of foods to eat.

It is best to eat whole foods in their natural form rather than processed, packaged, or prepared foods, which generally are not healthy and are full of empty calories, sugars, unhealthy fats, filler additives, over-processed grains, etc. While you may be accustomed to buying and eating packaged, prepared foods to save time, you will find it easy to toss together hearty vegetable salads with avocados, nuts, beans, and other healthy ingredients; fruit salads with yogurt and granola; stir-fries with salmon or tofu; and other easy-to-prepare dishes that you create yourself by mixing healthy foods. It's time to slip on the lab coat and provide you with some ideas for foods to pick up at your favorite grocery store, health food store, or farmer's market.

Examples of healthy foods to emphasize as part of your daily diet:

VEGETABLES: It is essential to make eating vegetables a daily priority. There are almost endless vegetables to choose from – some with funny names and shapes. Select from a variety of vegetables including spinach, broccoli, cabbage, cauliflower, chard, kale, mustard greens, turnips, rutabaga, carrots, beets, radishes, purple cabbage, parsley, asparagus, Brussels sprouts, red and green peppers, various sprouts including bean sprouts and alfalfa sprouts, sea vegetables, red lettuce, cucumbers, celery, asparagus, green beans, eggplant, scallions, onions, garlic, leeks, squash, pumpkin, snow peas, water chestnuts, and artichokes. If you don't have time to wash and prepare fresh vegetables, use pre-washed or frozen vegetables rather than canned. Also, when available, *buy organically grown vegetables*. Vegetables can also be consumed in the form of soups, stews, and fresh vegetable juices. (Juicing books have numerous suggestions for healthy vegetable juices.) It is best if you can make your own soups since most commercially prepared soups contain unhealthy additives. A second best alternative is to shop in a health food store or health-food section of a store for healthfully-prepared soups.

FRUIT: Eat a variety of fruits daily including grapefruit, oranges, tangerines, lemons, papaya, pineapple, mangos, blueberries, strawberries, raspberries, tomatoes, figs, apricots, peaches, plums, cherries, pears, cantaloupe, grapes, apples, avocados, and bananas. When available, *buy organically grown fruit*. You can also drink fresh low-sugar fruit juices, such as grapefruit juice. Fruits can be consumed in nutritional shakes and smoothies that are made from various fresh or frozen fruits including blueberries, strawberries, raspberries, peaches, and bananas, as well as soy or rice milk, wheat germ, organic yogurt, and vegetable, soy, or nut powders.

FATS: Healthy fats contain the essential and beneficial fatty acids and should be part of your daily diet. Foods rich in the important omega-3 fatty acids include flaxseed oil, fish oil, cold-water and fatty fish including salmon, tuna, cod, halibut, anchovy and shrimp, as well as fish oil or omega-3 supplements. Other sources of omega-3 fatty acids include pumpkin seeds, walnuts, canola oil, dark green leafy vegetables, sea vegetables, soybeans, wheat germ, and sprouts. If you don't eat fish several times a week, consider taking omega-3 fatty acid supplements or take one or two tablespoons of flaxseed oil daily. (Note: Store flaxseed oil in the refrigerator.)

Unprocessed olive oil and canola oil should be used as primary fats in your food preparation. Other beneficial fats are found in foods such as avocados, olives, nuts, seeds, and nut and seed butters. Good quality omega-6 fatty acids are found in raw nuts and seeds, legumes, and leafy green vegetables, evening primrose oil, borage oil, black currant seed oil, gooseberry oil, and grapeseed oil. Evening primrose or borage oil (found in health food stores) can be taken in the form of supplements. Avoid processed, hydrogenated grocery store vegetable oils such as corn, safflower, sunflower, soybean, cottonseed, and sesame oil as they contain transfats.

Nuts, seeds, and nut and seed butters contain both healthful fats and protein. There are a variety of nuts and seeds to choose from including almonds, pistachios, pecans, walnuts, cashews, hazelnuts, macadamia nuts, peanuts, natural peanut butter, almond butter, and tahini. Many nutritionists recommend raw nuts.

PROTEIN: It is important to eat adequate protein. Protein can be obtained from various foods including fish, nuts, seeds, nut and seed butters, tofu, beans, legumes, soybeans and soy foods such as tempeh, protein powder drinks, organic yogurt, and moderate amounts of animal protein such as organic cottage cheese and eggs. If you eat dairy, meat, or poultry, use only organic to avoid hormones, antibiotics, and meat or milk from animals fed chemicals or feed containing diseased or same-species meat.

Protein-containing foods that also provide complex carbohydrates include lentils, chickpeas, beans, legumes, peas, black beans, navy beans, lima beans, pinto beans, green beans, and wheat germ. Other foods that contain both proteins and complex carbohydrates include sprouts from grains, beans, lentils, seeds, vegetables, or alfalfa.

CARBOHYDRATES: Complex carbohydrate foods that can be part of a healthy diet include beans, peas and legumes, sprouted breads, brown rice, wild rice, basmati rice, unprocessed whole grains including buckwheat, millet, amaranth, quinoa, barley, rye, bulgur, wheat kernels, whole-grain pumpernickel, wheat grain, barley grain, cracked wheat, cracked wheat bread, corn, yams, oats, and whole-grain pasta. Try to limit processed carbohydrates. (Processed carbohydrates include muffins, pastries, sugary commercial breakfast cereals, pasta, white breads, rolls, and bagels, most crackers, cookies, cakes, and most prepared snacks, mixes, and convenience foods.)

SUPPLEMENTS: Multivitamin and mineral supplements are generally recommended by most doctors and nutritionists. If you are primarily a vegetarian, check with your doctor about taking additional vitamin-B12 and zinc supplements. Another important vitamin is vitamin D, which is found naturally in few foods except salmon and fatty fish, and is made when ultraviolet B from the Sun penetrates the skin. Certain foods, including milk and cereal, are also often fortified with some vitamin D. Because of the concern about skin cancer, many people may not be getting enough vitamin D. Inadequate amounts of vitamin D can cause rickets (soft bones, enlarged hearts) in babies and children, bone fractures in the elderly, and may be involved in cancer and autoimmune diseases. Vitamin D is also being evaluated for its antimicrobial properties, efficacy in fighting and reducing infections, including the flu,[45] and its association with a potentially lower risk of multiple sclerosis.[46] Vitamin D helps regulate calcium for bones, nerves, and heart, and currently recommended amounts may be inadequate.[47] Talk to your doctor about whether or not you need to supplement vitamin D as well what supplements you should be taking.

WATER: Drink at least 8 glasses of water a day. You can also drink herbal and green teas and mineral water. Avoid soft drinks and sugary drinks.

---

[45] FASEB Journal July 2005/Science News v. 170, No.20, 11/11/06

[46] JAMA v.296:2832-2838, 2006, http://jama.ama-assn.org/cgi/content/abstract/296/23/2832;;
J. of the American Dietetic Assoc 2006 03, v.106, Issue 3 http://www.adajournal.org/article/PIIS0002822305020845/pdf

[47] Science v. 302, No. 5652, p.1886, 12/12/03

How to Eat on 3:00 PM Days

You can begin getting accustomed to your scheduled *3:00 PM days* by not eating after 5:00 PM for several weeks, then work your way back to not eating after 4:30 PM, then 4:00 PM, then 3:30 PM, and finally 3:00 PM (or even earlier).

While it may seem unfathomable to not eat after 3:00 PM on your *3:00 PM days*, after several months you will find having a *rhythm* of *3:00 PM days* and *Free days* very easy to maintain. *It is easy to eat less on 3:00 PM days when you know you can eat more freely on Free days, and you are living in, or noticeably approaching, your ideal body.* While you should expect it to take several months to become comfortable with not eating after 3:00 PM, once you get used to it, you will realize you have found an easy way to achieve permanent weight control without endless and daily restriction from eating what you enjoy. You may be surprised to find that you feel better and sleep better on *3:00 PM days* without the burden of excess food. You can then awake to a healthy and substantial breakfast that will give you energy to meet the day. Eating most of your calories early in the day when you need the energy and will burn up what you consume is a healthy, satisfying strategy to control your weight. I suspect you will actually look forward to your *3:00 PM days*, and perhaps you will decide to have most of your days as *3:00 PM days* except for social occasions.

3:00 PM days should focus primarily on nutritious but tasty foods and drinks. The less food and fewer calories you eat, the more important it is that the food be highly nutritious and rich in essential amino acids found in protein, essential fatty acids found in high-quality fats and oils, and vitamins and minerals found in vegetables and other whole foods. On *3:00 PM days* you can select from the suggested foods listed in the previous section, while observing *The Ten Tips For Good Nutrition*. Concentrate on eating nutritious whole foods and include vegetables and fruits, along with protein and healthy fats. For example, on *3:00 PM days*, you can choose meals such as a salad with spinach, broccoli, sprouts, tofu, black beans, organic cottage cheese, fish, avocado, and olive oil; a fruit salad with grapefruit, strawberries, blueberries, raspberries, apples, granola, and organic yogurt; a grilled vegetable dish with almonds, wild rice, and tofu or salmon; or place fresh vegetables in an electric steamer with tempeh. You also may include vegetable juices and nutritious shakes. The idea is to supply all the nutrients you need without adding empty calories from foods that are processed, fried, or laden with sugar and empty calories.

If you find it difficult to eat less on some *3:00 PM days*, it may be helpful to obtain a portion of your nutrients in nutritious shakes, juices, and soups. Often people who have been eating in an unrestricted manner find it difficult to stop eating once they start. If you temper your eating by occasionally consuming a variety of foods and nutrients in the form of nutritious shakes, juices, or soups, you may be able to avoid the problem of not being able to stop eating once you start. When someone is addicted to cigarettes or alcohol and they decide to quit, they can just stop smoking cigarettes or drinking alcohol. When you want to control your weight, however, you can't just quit eating. Using soups, juices, and healthy shakes may help you to feel full before you have overeaten because liquids tend to fill up the stomach more quickly.

Nutritious shakes and smoothies can be made from ingredients like soy, vegetable and nut powders, organic yogurt, soymilk, rice milk, wheat germ, and fresh or frozen fruits including bananas, blueberries, strawberries, and peaches. Frozen fruit smoothies can be made thick and creamy. Fresh juices can be made with carrots, spinach, kale, beets, tomatoes, grapefruit, apples, or a combination of a variety of fruits and vegetables. Note that nutritional shakes do *not* include milkshakes and root-beer floats! Your shakes, smoothies, juices, and soups, however, can be delicious and satisfying. Eating whole foods such as fruits and vegetables that require little preparation can also be an effective tactic to avoid having to focus your attention on preparing elaborate meals. After all, *3:00 PM days* should focus on your life and your future, not on eating.

Following are three sample *3:00 PM day* menus. Remember to take supplements recommended by your doctor as well as omega-3 supplements (fish or flaxseed oil), and to drink plenty of water.

Sample Day 1

Breakfast: Granola with wheat germ, strawberries and rice milk, organic yogurt, and grapefruit juice.

Lunch: Salad with romaine, radishes, cauliflower, broccoli, cucumber, black beans, organic cottage cheese or tempeh, walnuts, turmeric, ginger, olive oil, lemon juice, and water or herbal tea.

2:30 PM Snack: Apple or orange, carrot sticks or a small handful of almonds, and water.

Sample Day 2

Breakfast: Oatmeal with soymilk and blueberries, seasonal fruit, and fresh vegetable juice.

Lunch: Pita bread stuffed with a mixture of albacore or wild salmon, a generous amount of spinach and plain organic yogurt, an apple, and water or herbal tea.

2:30 PM Snack: Pumpkin seeds, fresh carrot juice or dried fruit, and water.

Sample Day 3

Breakfast: Blueberry, banana, yogurt smoothie or organic scrambled eggs and fruit, whole-grain toast with almond butter, and green tea.

Lunch: Oven-roasted or stir fry vegetables with tofu, nuts, sesame seeds, olive oil, ginger, turmeric and other herbs, and water or herbal tea.

2:30 PM Snack: Vegetable juice, an orange, and water.

It may seem overwhelming to prepare whole, natural foods if you are in the habit of pulling a TV dinner out of the freezer or eating prepared processed foods. While new habits need to be formed, this should not be a difficult transition. It is helpful to keep healthy foods such as fruits, vegetables, whole grains, tofu or tempeh, organic yogurt, nuts, almond butter, salmon, albacore, and whole grain bread in your house and mix them together in various combinations for quick healthy breakfasts or salads and stir fries for lunches and *Free day* dinners. Experiment with various combinations of ingredients and have fun with preparing your own unique but simple recipes.

If you are accustomed to eating at night and are struggling on your *3:00 PM days*, you may find it satisfying to have a glass of soymilk or vegetable juice, a cup of clear soup, a cup of tea with milk in it, warm milk with nutmeg, or a piece of fruit. Having soymilk, soup, or juice may help soothe your stomach and take the edge off the desire to eat at night, and the liquid will help you feel less hungry. In addition, if you are going out at night on a *3:00 PM day*, you may want to have a glass of milk/soymilk, a small container of yogurt, or something similar before you leave to sustain your energy.

If after a few weeks you do not begin to feel your clothes getting looser and experience some weight loss, you can cut back on what you are consuming on *3:00 PM days*, especially empty calories. Alternatively, you may want to increase the number of *3:00 PM days* to at least six days per week and eat fairly lightly on any *Free day* evenings until you begin seeing positive results. *Free days* are most valuable for social dinners rather than an excuse to overeat. Remember, if you don't want to eat certain foods on *3:00 PM days*, then those foods should not be in your house tempting you.

Note: You should discuss this new eating style with your doctor and verify that he or she believes that not eating a meal between 3:00 PM and 6:00 AM five days a week is acceptable for you. Also, if you are on a special diet indicated by your doctor and your doctor gives you permission to not eat a meal after 3:00 PM, then eat your last meal by 3:00 PM on *3:00 PM days*.

How To Eat On Free Days

Free days should not only concentrate on nutrition, but also provide some pleasure eating in order to eliminate the feeling of endless deprivation. On *Free days* you can eat good nutritious foods in more generous amounts and later in the day. It is still important to be conscious of nutrition, and to limit sugar and junk foods. It is always a good idea to include nutritious foods from different groups, such as vegetables, fruits, fats, protein, and whole-food carbohydrates. However, on *Free days* you may mix in a few of your favorite foods, as long as they are reasonably nutritious. If you love to eat pasta, bagels, and even chocolate, then *Free days* are the days to eat them (in reasonable portions). As your weight comes under control and your body feels stronger and healthier from daily exercise and good nutrition, you can slowly wean yourself off most unhealthy foods containing sugar, processed carbohydrates, and unhealthy fats except for very special occasions. As your body becomes healthy and fit, it is likely that you will become less interested in putting unhealthy foods into it. *Free days* are most useful for social occasions when you are going out or having a dinner party with others. As the benefits of not eating at night begin to be obvious in your life, you may find you choose to eat most of your food early in the day even on many *Free days*.

There are various types of excellent, reasonably nutritious, and delightful foods you may choose to eat on *Free days*. They may include wonderful dishes based on Mediterranean, Japanese, Chinese, Mexican, Italian, Asian, or Indian cuisine. There are numerous healthy cookbooks that have delicious recipes. In addition to foods based on different regions of the world, you can make any type of recipe you enjoy including vegetable dishes, tofu dishes, rice dishes, bean dishes, pasta dishes, or your favorite fish. You also can make large salads with all your favorite ingredients, including spinach, broccoli and other vegetables, tempeh or tofu, black beans, organic cottage cheese or yogurt, salmon and other fish, olives, artichoke hearts, avocados, peppers, nuts, seeds, potatoes, olive oil, and any other food that lends itself to going into a salad.

Following is a sample *Free day* menu.

Sample Day

Breakfast: Whole grain cereal with rice milk, wheat germ, organic yogurt, fresh fruit, and apple juice.

Lunch: Salad with wild rice, red lettuce, tomatoes, avocado, water chestnuts, tofu, pecans, favorite spices, olive oil and lemon juice, an apple, and water or herbal tea.

Dinner: Vegetable stir-fry with rice noodles, olive oil, tamari sauce, almonds, sesame seeds, turmeric, ginger, and grilled salmon or tempeh, and water or herbal tea.

Certain individuals feel better with more protein and high-quality fats in their diets while others feel better eating more complex carbohydrate whole foods. The important factor in any diet is to get proper nutrition including the essential amino acids from protein foods, the essential omega-3 and omega-6 fatty acids, and monounsaturated fatty acids from foods such as nuts, seeds, fish, olive and flaxseed oil, as well as vitamins and minerals from fruits, vegetables, grains, and beans. In general, it is important to limit sugars, processed carbohydrates, and unhealthy fats (transfats).

For the first few weeks or months you may be tempted to overeat on *Free days*, but if you stick with this strategy you will eventually train your body and convince your subconscious mind to *know* that you will be able to eat more freely every few days as well as having a satisfying, healthy breakfast and lunch each day for the rest of your life, so *there is no need to ever overeat*. *3:00 PM days* may be challenging at first, but eventually you will feel better on *3:00 PM days* and look forward to them. The *3:00 PM/Free days* strategy works because you can eat more freely one or two days a week and still obtain and maintain the physique you choose.

A general note for eating: Don't sabotage yourself by buying low-fat or low-calorie versions of foods. Many low calorie foods are so awful that you may end up compensating by eating something really unhealthy that you would not have eaten if you had satisfied yourself by eating what you originally wanted. For example, if you happen to like cottage cheese, you are much better off eating a reasonable portion of regular organic cottage cheese that tastes good and satisfies you, rather than eating non-fat cottage cheese that tastes like cardboard and leaves you so unsatisfied you make up for it by either piling something frightful on top of it to mask the taste or by eating a gallon of ice cream after you finish the calorie-saving cottage cheese. Eat a reasonable amount of the "real thing" that satisfies you and be happy, so you don't end up compensating with something worse. "Low-fat" foods are also often filled with sugar, transfats, and other unhealthy fillers.

Note: If you are on a special diet indicated by your doctor, you should stick to the foods specified by your diet.

Introduction to Appendix 1:
Essential Nutrients and Where to Find Them

Why does it seem that grocery stores are filled with foods that are somewhat or even completely unhealthy? Perhaps because that's what consumers ask for by what they choose to buy. Shoppers see boxes, jars, and cans of food lining the shelves and assume the foods inside are reasonably nutritious, so they shop for taste and price. Unfortunately, most of the processed and packaged foods are full of sugars, unhealthy fats, and a myriad of ingredients our bodies were never designed to consume or use. People also tend to follow eating and grocery-shopping habits they learned from parents, yet hope to avoid looking like their parents. Each of us is responsible for making wise lifestyle choices as adults, and not continuing unhealthy family traditions.

When a person actually makes an effort to put nutrients into his or her body and avoid sugar, transfats, bleached flour, hormones, fillers, pesticides, etc., he or she will often have to spend more money. It often costs more to purchase a healthier version of a food, such as organic fruits, vegetables, and dairy, and people just are not sure that buying organic foods offers enough of a guarantee that they can escape cancer or other diseases by avoiding pesticides, growth hormones, antibiotics and other chemicals that are liberally pumped into mainstream food sources. Fruit juice is another example of higher cost being associated with making a healthier choice. Have you noticed that buying a fruit juice made up of the actual juice named on the label rather than a mixture of diluted cheaper juices and one or more varieties of sugar (corn syrup, dextrose, sucrose, fructose, cane juice, and artificial sweeteners) cost two to four times more?

When comparing other foods such as apples to potato chips, however, it is usually less expensive to eat an apple for a snack than a bag of potato chips. Fresh fruits and vegetables as a group are often less expensive than processed foods. If you are reading this book, odds are you are eating more food than your body requires, so if you buy smaller amounts of high quality and nutritious foods that sometimes cost more than unhealthy alternatives, the total dollars spent on food will be about the same. Besides, by not filling your shopping cart with unneeded junk foods, you are saving money.

I strongly believe, however, it is worth spending extra for nutritious foods when a nutritious food cost more than its less healthy counterpart. I often compare the few cents to few dollars spent on a healthy version of a food to the hundreds or thousands it may be saving me in medical costs for some illness resulting from the accumulative toxic effects of eating unhealthy foods. There is sufficient evidence that the hormones and pesticides in non-organic animal and plant foods can cause cancer. For example, women with elevated levels of pesticides in their breast tissue have a greater breast cancer risk.[48] In addition, high levels of circulating IGF-I (a growth factor released in cows when they are injected with bovine growth hormone) are associated with increased risk of several common cancers, including those of the prostate, breast, colorectum, and lung.[49] And it's not just the monetary cost since the effect of illness on one's life is immeasurable. While occasionally eating small amounts of the harmful substances contained in most processed and non-organic foods is unlikely to have a significant negative effect on one's health, the eventual accumulation of harmful substances put into one's body day after day adds up and can have substantial unwanted consequences.

Another reason people don't choose healthy foods over cheaper, more prevalent, easy to find, processed foods containing pesticides, hormones, sugars, and fillers, is that we all have heard of the example of the guy who did everything wrong – drank, smoked, never exercised, ate junk food – and lived to 99; or the woman athlete who seemed to do everything right in terms of nutrition, exercise, sleep, etc., and developed cancer and died at 35. These extreme examples allow people to rationalize avoiding regular exercise and eating poorly. There is another category of folks who tell themselves they eat healthfully when they really don't, and pretend walking twenty feet from their car to their front door constitutes exercise.

A rational approach to making food choices is to take steps to increase your odds of a healthy life by educating yourself about basic nutritional principles, which I have endeavored to include in this chapter as well as in *Appendix 1: Essential Nutrients and Where to Find Them*. It is sensible to practice good nutritional habits by making a lot of small wise eating choices. In conjunction with making daily smart food choices, we can choose to exercise for ten minutes as detailed in Chapter 4, and choose to get adequate sleep as discussed in Chapter 5. I look at each choice I make in favor of a nutritious food rather than an unhealthy food as one small step in the direction of health

---

[48] http://www.mayoclinic.com/health/breast-cancer-prevention/WO00091

[49] Journal of the National Cancer Institute v.93, No.3, p.238, 2/7/01; Lancet v.351, No.9113, p.1393, 5/9/98; Journal of the National Cancer Institute v.92, No.18, p.1472, 9/20/00

and vitality. The way I see it, the accumulation of good food choices, decisions to exercise, and getting adequate sleep stack the odds in favor of a long, vital, and healthy life. Occasionally, if I eat a cookie or skip exercise for a couple of days, it is unlikely to have a huge impact on my health and well-being as long as ninety-five percent of the time I make good choices. I should mention that well-being is greatly enhanced when one looks in the mirror and sees a strong, fit body and feels the results of healthy food choices. A strong body and clear mind are your means to pursuing and accomplishing your dreams.

Making wise food choices and having a healthy lifestyle can make a difference in your body's ability to resist and recover from illness and disease. This was emphasized in a study reported several years ago in *Journal of the American Medical Association* in a concluding statement: "substantial evidence indicates that diets using nonhydrogenated unsaturated fats as the predominant form of dietary fat, whole grains as the main form of carbohydrates, an abundance of fruits and vegetables, and adequate omega-3 fatty acids can offer significant protection against coronary heart disease." The researchers also pointed out that combining this type of a diet with regular physical activity, avoiding smoking, and maintaining a healthy body weight may prevent the majority of cardiovascular disease in Western populations.[50] While there are genetic and environmental factors beyond our control and we can't absolutely prevent disease, we can increase the odds of having a healthier body by nutritious eating, exercise, and sleep.

The sections in Appendix 1 explain why it is so important to eat the types of foods listed in *The Ten Tips for Good Nutrition* and *What Foods to Emphasize on 3:00 PM Days and Free Days*. Appendix 1 also highlights many surprising findings of nutrition research, as well as why our bodies need protein, fats, fruits, and vegetables. The information is intended as a reference and guide to assist you in sorting out the food choices that work best for you. The contents of the *Appendix 1: Essential Nutrients and Where to Find Them*, which begins on page 117, are as follows:

---

[50] JAMA v.288, No.20, p.2569, 11/27/02

Before delving deeper into nutrition, it's time to leave our stomachs behind and move on with the rest of the story.

Chapter 4

The Ten-Minute Maximized Workout

Make it quick, easy, and convenient.

This exercise strategy is based on getting ten minutes of convenient, muscle-building exercise six days a week.

Note: Talk to your doctor before starting any exercise program, especially if you have health problems or have not exercised for a long time.

"Hey Isabelle, looks like we're the only fools working late again."
Isabelle seemed to meet Jane only in the copy room, yet they had pieced together a friendship from snippets of conversation.

"It's becoming the norm," Isabelle answered with a wry smile.

"I wouldn't mind, but it keeps me from getting to the gym in the evening. I had made a New Year's resolution to exercise an hour a day, and in the past few months I've only managed to go a few times. I hate it when I can't exercise!" Jane turned from the copy machine giving Isabelle her full attention.

"I made a New Year's resolution to exercise too. I rarely miss a day." Isabelle looked happy and relaxed even at the end of a long workday.

"Yeah, it shows. But how do you manage it? You're as busy as I am." Jane looked frustrated.

"It's no big deal. I invested about $50 at a garage sale and installed my mini health club in a corner of my bedroom. My exercise is a 10-minute detour from my morning primping routine. It's really quick and convenient!" Isabelle smiled.

"Isabelle, where do you get all your good ideas?" Jane smiled back.

Jane and Isabelle both wanted to exercise every day. Jane's New Year's resolution had been for an hour a day and was impractical with her busy life. Isabelle had made her New Year's resolution to exercise ten minutes a day six days a week for the whole year and beyond. At the rate she was going Jane would have time to exercise sporadically at best until she got frustrated and gave up, while Isabelle would be able to exercise ten minutes six days a week all year, each and every year for the foreseeable future. Who is better off?

Why is it important to exercise at all? Most people have heard that exercise is important and that it provides many health benefits including weight control. Exercise offers numerous other benefits in addition to weight control that enhance the quality of life. A few of these benefits are that exercise: improves memory and cognitive ability; improves the cardiovascular system; improves posture; reduces the risk of falling and the resulting fractured or broken bones; increases energy level, strength, endurance, balance, flexibility, and muscle tone; helps ward off osteoporosis by maintaining bone density; relieves depression; raises self-esteem; reduces the risk of heart disease, stroke, diabetes, and many other diseases; improves sleep; increases the blood vessels in and the blood supply to the brain enabling us to think better; increases levels of chemicals and growth factors in the brain that are involved in motor function, cognition, reasoning, thinking, and learning, and that are believed to prevent the connections between nerve cells from breaking down and also help them grow back, as well as reducing Alzheimer's disease risk; and reduces age-related disability characterized by generalized weakness, impaired mobility and balance, poor endurance, and loss of muscle strength, which dramatically affect our chances of living an independent life as we age. Seems pretty convincing to me.

Why Ten Minutes and Not Thirty To Sixty Minutes?

I am not implying that thirty to sixty minutes is not better than ten minutes, but most people can't find (or don't want to find) thirty to sixty minutes for exercise every day. Therefore, a commitment to ten minutes is a good compromise, as it may result in more total exercise over time. The ten-minute strategy is aimed at those of us who, even if we would like to exercise thirty to sixty minutes a day, never find time. Thirty to sixty minutes for exercise is a large chunk of time out of an already busy day and often seems too overwhelming. Even though some of us may have good intentions about exercise, we never quite manage to do it. Whether you do or don't want to exercise, given the numerous important benefits to your quality of life and weight control success, you may concede to ten minutes.

This exercise strategy employs the psychology of promising yourself, "If I will just do ten minutes of exercise every day, that is sufficient, and I promise I will not exceed that ten minutes or make myself feel guilty about not doing more." This will allow you to get into a pattern of daily exercise that is not something you will continually make excuses not to do because you don't have time or it is too much of a hassle. Absolutely everyone can manage to take ten minutes out of each day as long as their exercise location is so convenient that there is no extra time required for travel and they don't have to dress in special clothing.

By exercising ten minutes every day you can get into a daily pattern of exercise. If you want to do something more, then add some aerobic exercise (walking, cycling, swimming, jogging, etc.) at a different time of day, but don't upset the psychology of, "I only have to do this quick workout for ten minutes." It is important to convince your subconscious mind that you really will only do your 10 minutes and no more, otherwise you will constantly find excuses why you don't have time to work out on any given day. If you are not already a consistent exerciser, then it may be beneficial not to extend your workout beyond 10 minutes or your subconscious mind will know that you have not really made a commitment to only 10 minutes and it may become resistant to doing any exercise at all.

To illustrate this, here is an analogy of you and your subconscious – you are the mother and your subconscious is your son: The mother wants her son to go to the bank with her every day to deposit cash from her small business, which will take about 10 minutes. If she only makes him go to the bank each day and therefore affirms to him that that is all he will have to do, he is happy to go along. If she starts adding other errands to their bank trips, such as a 20 minute stop at the grocery store or a 15 minute stop at the post office, he will eventually become resistant to going with her at all. He will begin to dread even just going to the bank and will not trust her when she says "we are only going to the bank", because she has already demonstrated to him that "going to the bank" may also mean other time-consuming and boring stops. It is important to limit your exercise time and get yourself into a habit or routine that you are comfortable doing every day (actually only six days a week). If you know it is only for 10 minutes, you are more likely to do it.

If you can't squeeze ten minutes of exercise in during the morning or evening, then do five minutes in the morning and five minutes in the evening. You can split the workout that you are going to do on a given day in half or even spread it out throughout the day if it is absolutely necessary. Just get the exercises done six days a week.

If you already do thirty to sixty minutes of exercise or go to a gym every day to work out, it fits into your schedule, and you enjoy it, great! Just make sure you are getting a total-body strength-training workout along with any aerobics you may be doing. The 10-minute *exercise strategy* described in this book is geared toward the average person who has not found a successful exercise program and needs the benefits of strength training.

Why Muscle-Building, Weight-Training?

Weight training is also referred to as strength training, resistance training, or weight-bearing exercise, and involves lifting, moving, pulling, or pushing against resistance or weight. Weight training will cause you to replace fat tissue with muscle tissue, which will increase your body's metabolism twenty-four hours a day. Increasing muscle tissue will allow you to burn more calories even while you are not exercising because muscle is active tissue and burns more calories than fat tissue. Men can usually lose weight and body fat faster and easier than women because men generally have more muscle mass and therefore burn more calories. Weight-bearing exercise will also improve your balance, endurance, strength, and posture, and help ward off osteoporosis by maintaining or restoring bone density. Weight lifting will also help push back other deleterious effects of aging that can make you become frail and weak as you age. Having a strong, muscular body will make you feel more empowered, more attractive, and more self-confident.

Focusing your exercise on weight lifting will not only give you a stronger, healthier body, but will enable you to redistribute your weight and give you a more balanced physique. Although we see professional body builders redistribute their weight by building muscle in their shoulders, arms, back, and legs, while toning and trimming down their abdomen and hips, we often don't think that we can redistribute our own weight to better balance and strengthen our bodies. Many people are born with puny arms and shoulders, but after proper weight training can balance their naturally stronger legs with a strong upper body. Strengthening all the major muscle groups from arms and shoulders through back and abdomen to buttocks and legs, will balance your entire physique. Weight training is also a way for someone who is obese to manage exercise without the pounding of jogging or aerobics.

According to researchers, as humans age beyond 40, approximately one-third to one-half of a pound of muscle is lost each year and replaced by fat. This contributes to a loss of about one to two percent of strength each year.[51] As muscles weaken and movement becomes more difficult, people eventually become more sedentary and dependent. This apparent dismal inevitability of our aging bodies can actually be slowed and reversed by strength training. In fact, high-intensity resistance exercise training has been shown to be a feasible and effective means to counteract muscle weakness and physical

---

[51] Miriam Nelson, Ph.D. Tufts University, www.strongwomen.com

frailty in very elderly people. In a study, one-hundred frail nursing home residents with an average age of 87 increased their muscle strength by 113 percent after 10 weeks of resistance exercise training.[52] Researchers have studied the effects of weight training by having older adults move their muscles against a resistance, or weight, and then slowly and progressively increase the amount of weight moved or lifted. The results showed that the bodies of older adults can rebuild lost muscle mass just like younger bodies. The researchers documented some of the benefits of strength training, which include: (1) an increase in balance and flexibility; (2) a reduction in fractures and broken bones; (3) a reduction in bone loss and restoration of bone density; (4) an increase in physical activity and vitality; (5) a leaner, more muscular body having a higher metabolic rate thereby enhancing weight control; (6) an improvement in depression and self-esteem; (7) a relief in symptoms of osteoarthritis and rheumatoid arthritis; (8) a reduction in the risk of heart disease and diabetes; (9) an improvement in sleep; and (10) the ability of overweight people to become stronger and more physically active.[53] We are not destined to become weaker and weaker with each passing decade, but can remain vital and strong throughout our lives.

Engaging in exercise also increases the blood vessels in your brain, which will help you to think better. As discussed in Chapter 6, *Successful Aging*, in the section on *Exercise and Aging*, the *brain* is enhanced through exercise. Not only does exercise increase the vasculature and blood supply to the brain, but there are chemicals and growth factors in the brain whose levels are raised from exercise.[54] These chemicals or neurotrophic factors that are released from nerve cells during exercise help nerve cells resist illness or injury, prompt them to grow and multiply, and strengthen connections between nerve cells. One of these chemicals, called Brain Derived Growth Factor, is believed to prevent the connections between nerve cells from breaking down and also help them grow back. Not only do these chemicals promote learning and memory, but may also help the brain resist Alzheimer's and Parkinson's diseases.[55] There are several of these brain chemicals that are protective to neurons including Brain Derived Neurotrophic Factor and other neurotrophins and growth factors, which are believed to promote the survival and differentiation of neurons and promote plasticity of nerves and synapses.[56] In fact, studies have shown that exercise increases the levels of

---

[52] New England Journal of Medicine v.330, No.25, 1769, 6/23/94

[53] Strong Women Stay Young, Miriam Nelson, 4/4/2000

[54] The Journal of Neuroscience v.20, No.8, p.2926, 4/15/00

[55] Science News v.169, No.8, p.122, 2/25/06; Stealing Time: The New Science of Aging, Warshofsky TV Books 1999 p.222

[56] Science v.295, No.5560, 3/102, p.1651-53, 1729-34; Science v.270, No.5236, 10/2795, p.593

certain growth factors in the areas of the brain involved in motor function, cognition, reasoning, thinking, and learning. When groups of healthy people of the same age were compared by a battery of cognitive tests, the groups that exercised performed better cognitively than the groups that did not exercise.[57]

It simply makes sense to strengthen, tone, and increase our muscle mass. Imagine a model of a human skeleton. Perhaps you remember one hanging from a stand in your science class when you were in school. Picture this skeleton with a bunch of rubber organs attached to it with tape in their proper places. Then add Saran wrap to simulate skin. How can this skeleton possibly hold itself up without being suspended from something? If you unhook it from its stand, it will collapse on the floor under gravity. What is keeping our bodies from collapsing under gravity? The answer is our muscles. Think about your own skeleton, organs, skin, blood, etc. The only way you can stand, move, run, sit, climb, and get yourself up is by using your muscles. It makes sense that having more muscle tissue and stronger muscles will make holding your body up with good posture and moving it around much easier. Strong muscles will take strain off your skeleton!

If you embrace weight training, you will be able to raise your overall metabolism by reducing fat tissue and increasing lean muscle tissue, reshape your body, get stronger, burn fat, improve your balance, and maintain or replace the muscle tissue that is naturally lost during aging. Weight-training exercise will allow men and women to replace bulky fat tissue with lean muscle tissue. Most women as well as men need to build muscles in their arms and upper body. Even people who regularly exercise often do not build their arms, chest, and backs. They often end up with noodle arms, puny shoulders, protruding abdomens, and slouched posture. If you follow the exercises described in this chapter, you can easily redistribute your weight to balance your body musculature by lifting weights using all your main muscle groups. Weight lifting is also an exercise that can provide nearly instant gratification for the effort put into it. After just a few weeks of working out, you can actually see the muscles you are targeting begin to get bigger and more defined. After a few months, your body will become firmer and begin to reshape. You will be able to see muscles develop in your arms, shoulders, chest, back and legs, while you are trimming and strengthening your whole body. It is extremely gratifying! In addition, if you go through the weight-

---

[57] Stealing Time: The New Science of Aging, Warshofsky TV Books 1999 p.222-223/ Nature, 373, 109 Cotman 1995

lifting routines described in this chapter rapidly without taking significant rests, you will get an aerobic-like workout as well.

For Those Averse to Lifting Weights or Who Desire Aerobics

Aerobic exercise has enormously important benefits, and if you are currently running, cycling, hiking, or taking a class for cardiovascular health, you should continue. Perhaps you can add weight training to your aerobic exercise in order to create balanced muscle mass and strength. Aerobic exercise is good for your cardiovascular system and can help you lose weight because you are burning calories during exercise. If you wish to include aerobic exercise in your workout, it is acceptable to replace two or three ten-minute weight-training workouts with vigorous aerobic workouts each week. *If you are averse to weigh lifting entirely*, you can still do the daily workout using a resistance-providing aerobic exercise machine for ten to twenty minutes instead of weights. Examples of resistance-providing aerobic exercise equipment include a Nordic Trac, a rowing machine, an elliptical, a stair climber, a stepper, an exercise bike, or an incline treadmill. If you are substituting the "ten-minute workout" with aerobic exercise, it is beneficial to use resistance-providing aerobic exercise equipment vigorously for at least ten to twenty minutes.

A strong body contributes to making a strong mind and a strong person who is more resistant to mental and physical stress. Allowing your body to unnecessarily deteriorate can cause a general deterioration in other aspects of your life.

Why Must Exercise Be Convenient?

It is important to make your exercise workout convenient so that you don't need to go anywhere special to do it. Placing a few pieces of exercise equipment in a convenient location and only exercising ten minutes a day, lowers the psychological activation barrier to performing daily exercise. Years ago I had a friend whose father was a physician with a busy lifestyle. He managed to get exercise every day by putting an exercise bike and hand weights in his bathroom. Each morning when he got out of bed he headed for the bathroom where he rode his bike for 10 minutes and then jumped in the shower. He could then dress, go downstairs to eat breakfast, and be on his way. He didn't sabotage himself by thinking, "Well, I really should get at least 30 minutes of exercise rather than 10 minutes". This would have set him up for failure because he really didn't have 30 minutes to spare and may have skipped exercising all together.

Everyone can get up 10 minutes earlier, but 30 minutes may contribute to sleep deprivation. This doctor was successful because he kept his exercise equipment someplace extremely convenient while limiting his exercise time. If he had to go to a gym, or even to the other end of the house, it would have been easy to skip his 10-minute workout. But with his exercise equipment situated between the toilet and the shower, it was pretty hard to avoid. Also, he had a beautiful mural on the bathroom wall with a nature setting that he could look at while taking his ride. His secret was limiting his exercise time to something he could not make an excuse not to do, and locating his equipment in a place that was too convenient to avoid.

You may think that going to a gym 4 or 5 days a week would be a great way to get fit, but when it comes down to it, you may not really want to go or have the time. Use the money you would spend on a gym contract to purchase weights and a bench, and spend the rest on a new wardrobe. It is a lot more convenient to spend ten minutes lifting weights on your way to the shower in the morning than driving to the gym on your lunch hour or after work and having to change clothes, face the crowd, then shower again, and drive back to work or home. Make your workout routine fast and convenient. If you are fortunate enough to live or work conveniently close to a gym and you enjoy going there, then you can do this workout or something similar in the gym using their equipment.

Place your bench and weights someplace in your house you can't avoid. (See equipment in next section.) If you want to listen to the radio or watch the news during your workout, then put your equipment nearby. You should keep a pair of athletic shoes next to your weights so you can quickly pull them on as you begin your daily workout. Also, regarding convenience, wear anything you are comfortable in: a tee-shirt, shorts, stretch pants, night shirt, etc. It is also beneficial to view yourself in a mirror to check your form.

The secret to making yourself work out every day is limiting your exercise time to something you can't make an excuse not to do, and locating your equipment in a place that is too convenient to avoid.

The Workout – Daily Exercises

Getting into a successful pattern of doing daily exercise involves managing your mind. If it takes too long or requires too much effort, you probably won't be able to stick with it. The idea is to get the most out of the time you spend each day working out. It is important to set an easy, short workout plan *and follow it.* (It's time to change out of the lab coat into gym shorts and shoes!)

Equipment

The only *equipment* required is *dumbbell weights, ankle weights,* and a standard *exercise weight-lifting bench* or equivalent.

A *weight bench,* or equivalent, is required for two of the upper body exercises (Exercise 9: CHEST—FLYE and Exercise 10: CHEST—PRESS) and one of the lower body exercises (Exercise 5: QUADRICEPS—SITTING LEG EXTENSION). Note that a more sophisticated weight bench can be purchased having a built in leg-extension and leg-curl mechanism for doing lower body Exercise 5: QUADRICEPS—EXTENSION and Exercise 6: HAMSTRING—CURLS.

Dumbbells are small weights you hold in each hand. If you are new to weight lifting, you will begin with a set of low-weight dumbbells, such as 3 or 5 pounds depending on your strength. You should be able to lift the dumbbells over your head easily, but with some effort. As you progress, you will want to increase the weight you lift and will need higher-weight dumbbells, maybe 5 or 8 pounds. Over time, you should be able to increase the amount of weight you lift and may eventually need higher weight dumbbell sets. You can also purchase adjustable dumbbells that can be adjusted from approximately 3 pounds up to approximately 50 pounds. The majority of exercises described use dumbbell weights.

Ankle weights are weights that can be strapped around each ankle and usually range from 1 pound to 20 pounds. If you are new to weight lifting, you will begin with a set of low-weight ankle weights, such as 3 or 5 pounds depending on your strength. You can purchase adjustable ankle weights that adjust from 1 pound to 5 pounds, 1 pound to 10 pounds, 1 pound to 15 pounds, or 1 pound to 20 pounds. The ankle weights are used for lower body

Exercises 6: HAMSTRING—CURLS and may also be used for Exercise 5: QUADRICEPS—EXTENSION (unless you have a special weight bench with a built in leg-extension and leg-curl mechanism).

Definitions

SETS: A *set* is a group of repetitions (the number of times you lift and lower a weight) that you do without resting. The exercise strategy described in this book consists of doing 1 set of each exercise. Advanced weight lifters may decide to do 2 sets or possibly 3 sets of each exercise.

REPETITIONS: *Repetitions* are the number of times you lift and lower your weights within a set. For example, you may be doing one set consisting of 12 repetitions of each of the weight lifting exercises described below. One repetition generally involves moving your weights, or all or part of your body, from its starting position up to its high position and back down to the starting position. In a squat or lunge, the repetition involves moving your entire body, along with the weights, down to a low position then back up to the starting position.

BREATHING: When a body builder is lifting a heavy weight, it is generally recommended that he or she breathe out during the lifting phase and breathe in during the lowering phase. However, when you are doing this workout and moving quickly and smoothly through an exercise faster than your natural rhythm of *breathing*, then breathe normally so that you don't increase the rate you breathe too much and hyperventilate. *It is very important to keep breathing and not to hold your breath, which you may find yourself doing inadvertently.*

Stretching

Every day you need to stretch. It is best to stretch during your workout time, but if it is not possible, you can easily fit it in sometime during the day or evening. Here are three stretches you should do every day:

1. Sit on the floor with your legs straight in front of you. While keeping your legs and back straight, lean forward and reach for and hold onto (if you can) your toes. Hold it for a count of 100.

2. Sit on the floor and spread your legs to the sides as far as possible. While keeping your legs and back straight, reach toward your right foot, and hold your toes (if you can) for a count of 100. Then reach for your left foot and hold it for a count of 100.

3. Stretch your calves one at a time. Stand up with the ball of one foot resting on a thick book and the heel of that same foot on the floor. Hold it for the count of 100. Switch to the other leg and do the same.

The Workout

I have included descriptions and pictures of *20* weight-lifting routines that are split in half giving you *10* upper-body routines one day and *10* lower-body routines the second day, which you should alternate every other day for 6 days out of each week. Weight lifting should focus on the upper body one day and the lower body the next day so that you are not working the same muscle groups two days in a row. This is important because during weight training your muscles are being stressed and overloaded, then when you are not working these muscles, they rebuild, grow, and strengthen themselves. It is important that you give your muscles time to rebuild and strengthen.

The routines in this book were chosen to enable you to build and strengthen the muscles in your chest, shoulders, biceps, triceps, back, thighs, hips/buttocks, abdomen, and calves. According to many weight-training experts, achieving a full development and reshaping of your body requires what is called *muscle isolation* in which you focus on working one muscle group at a time by doing several different exercises on that muscle group. In order to limit the workout to ten minutes, we will not have enough time to do the number of sets required to achieve the level of muscle isolation described by professional weight lifters. However, we will do a couple of different exercises on each of the primary muscle groups and you will be able to slowly redistribute your weight and noticeably reshape your body as you increase the amount of weight you lift.

The amount of time you spend working out each day can be varied by the length of time you rest between exercises as well as how many repetitions you do of each exercise. In the beginning the 1-Set workout (described below) may take 15 minutes or more while you learn the exercises. Eventually, you will be able to move smoothly and rapidly through the exercises fast enough to get through them in 10 minutes. You are way ahead by doing a 1-Set workout indefinitely and consistently six days a week rather than occasionally doing a longer workout.

Moving rapidly through your exercises will also give you a short, focused, intense aerobic-like workout especially if you do more repetitions. Be careful to make your movements smooth and concentrated with a brief pause at the top and bottom of each lift. In the beginning, you will need to give yourself time to learn and get accustomed to the exercises. *If you are short of time or tired on any particular day, do fewer repetitions of each exercise rather than skipping your workout entirely.*

It is a good idea to begin using weights that are reasonably light. Nevertheless, in order to progress and continue to replace fat tissue with muscle tissue, you will need to gradually increase the weights that you use. You will build stronger muscles by using heavier weights. You do not need to worry about "bulking up" and looking like a professional body builder unless you spend hours in a gym every day. Increasing the weight you lift, along with the number of repetitions, will allow you to continue to improve your body.

Muscle is stimulated during both the lifting and lowering of a weight, so concentrate on moving smoothly and deliberately in both directions through the entire repetition. It is better to cut back the number of repetitions rather than inadequately completing the full movement. Also, it is important to realize that some muscle soreness is normal, but injury is not normal. When you begin exercising, you can expect that the muscles you work one day may be somewhat sore the next day, especially when you start new exercises. Soreness means you are developing your muscles. But an injury will set you back and slow your progress significantly. So challenge yourself when you work out, but don't push yourself beyond your limit. You should not push until the muscles you are working experience pain.

Alternative to Weight Lifting

As mentioned in the above subsection, *For Those Averse to Lifting Weights or Who Desire Aerobics*, if you wish to include **aerobic exercise** in your workout, you can substitute two or three aerobic days each week. *If you are averse to weigh lifting entirely*, you can still do the daily workout using a resistance-providing aerobic exercise machine for ten to twenty minutes instead of weights. Examples of ***resistance-providing aerobic exercise equipment*** include a Nordic Trac, a rowing machine, an elliptical, a stair climber, a stepper, an exercise bike, or an incline treadmill. If you are substituting the "ten-minute workout" with aerobic exercise, it is preferable to use resistance-providing aerobic exercise equipment vigorously for ten to twenty minutes.

Note: If you are new to weight training, you may want to schedule an appointment with a professional trainer or expert to help you begin your 10-minute workout plan. A trainer can also help you get started with the proper level of dumbbell weights you should begin with, and show you how to properly lift them. In addition, you should talk to your doctor about this program if you are new to weight lifting and have any health concerns.

The "1-Set" Workout

- Do 1 set of each of the **10** exercises (either upper body or lower body) that are specified for a given day. The exercises are described in detail beginning on page 66 below.

- If you are new to weight lifting, begin with only 1 or 2 repetitions, then 4 or 5 repetitions for each exercise, then work up to 12 repetitions for each exercise.

- If you are new to weight lifting, begin with light weights with which you feel comfortable: perhaps 3 pounds or 5 pounds.

- For each day's **10** exercises you will do:

  1 Set consisting of 12 repetitions using weights appropriate for your strength and size.

- As you get used to the daily exercise, you should be able to do this 1-Set workout comfortably in 10 minutes. If you are not making it in 10 minutes, then shorten your rests between exercises or reduce the number of repetitions. Be careful to make your movements smooth and concentrated, flexing and contracting the muscles being worked.

- Continue with this workout indefinitely and increase the weight you lift as needed. You can increase the number of repetitions to 14, 16, or 18, which will give you a more vigorous workout.

2-Set or 3-Set Workouts for Advanced Weight Lifters

Note: If you are already an *advanced* weight lifter, you may do a 2-Set or a 3-Set workout. The exercises are described in detail beginning on page 66 below.

- The instructions are the same as the 1-Set workout except that you will do 2 or 3 sets of each different exercise that is specified for a given day.

- For a **2-Set workout** do 10 to 12 repetitions using low weights for Set 1, and 8 to 10 repetitions using higher weights for Set 2.

    Set 1:   Low weights   10 to 12 repetitions
    Set 2:   High weights   8 to 10 repetitions

- For a **3-Set workout** you can use three different dumbbell weight sets – low, medium, and high. For each exercise you can do three sets:

    Set 1:   Low weights   10 to 12 repetitions
    Set 2:   Medium weights   8 to 10 repetitions
    Set 3:   High weights   6 to 8 repetitions

- If you do the two or three set workouts in close to 10 minutes you will get an aerobic-like workout along with the weight training. If you are not able to get through the two sets in close to 10 minutes, then go back to the 1-Set workout with 12 to 18 repetitions.

Alternate Upper-Body and Lower-Body Exercises

There are 10 upper-body exercises and 10 lower-body exercises. You will alternate "upper-body day" exercises and "lower-body day" exercises so that, for example:

Monday will be	**10** upper-body exercises
Tuesday will be	**10** lower-body exercises
Wednesday will be	**10** upper-body exercises
Thursday will be	**10** lower-body exercises
Friday will be	**10** upper-body exercises
Saturday will be	**10** lower-body exercises
Sunday will be	A rest day with enjoyable activities.

It is helpful, especially in the beginning, to exercise in front of a mirror so you can check your form.

Please see the *Cut-Out Pages* of the *Daily Workout Summary* at the end of the book.

UPPER-BODY EXERCISES

Note: Using weights that are too heavy can cause poor form or injury, so make sure you are using weights that challenge your muscles without straining them. If possible, stand in front of a mirror to monitor your movements. Remember to use the *Cut-Out Pages* of the *Daily Workout Summary* at the end of the book as a daily reference once you are more familiar with the exercises.

The following upper-body exercises are described in detail below:

Exercise 1:   BICEPS--CURL
Exercise 2:   BICEPS--HAMMER CURL

Exercise 3:   SHOULDERS--SIDE RAISE
Exercise 4:   SHOULDERS--OVERHEAD PRESS

Exercise 5:   BACK--BENT LIFT
Exercise 6:   BACK--UPRIGHT ROW

Exercise 7:   TRICEPS--EXTENSIONS
Exercise 8:   TRICEPS--PUSHBACK

Exercise 9:   CHEST--FLYE
Exercise 10: CHEST--BENCH PRESS

Exercise 1: BICEPS--CURL

Equipment: Dumbbell weights.

For each repetition:

Stand up straight with feet about shoulder-width apart and abdominal muscles tightened. Avoid locking knees. Remember to keep breathing, don't hold your breath, and when possible exhale as you lift weights.

<u>Start/Finish</u> position: Hold dumbbells down close to your sides and slightly in front of your thighs with palms facing forward.

Keeping your upper arms stationary, bend elbows and raise dumbbells up to your shoulders in an arc-motion so that your palms are facing your shoulders in the <u>Midpoint</u> position. Pause briefly.

Lower dumbbells back down in an arc-motion to <u>Start/Finish</u> position.

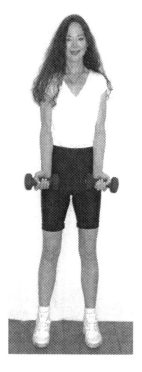

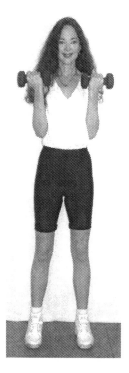

<u>Start/Finish</u> position   **<u>Midpoint</u> position**

Exercise 2: BICEPS--HAMMER CURL

Equipment: Dumbbell weights.

For each repetition:

Stand up straight with feet about shoulder-width apart and abdominal muscles tightened. Avoid locking knees. Remember to keep breathing, don't hold your breath, and when possible exhale as you lift weights.

Start/Finish position: Hold dumbbells straight down close to your sides with palms facing inward toward the outside of your thighs.

Keeping your upper arm stationary and your palms facing inward, bend right elbow and raise right dumbbell up to your right shoulder in an arc-motion to the Midpoint position. Pause briefly.

Lower right dumbbell back down in an arc-motion to Start/Finish position.

Repeat with left dumbbell: Keeping your upper arm stationary and your palms facing inward, bend left elbow and raise left dumbbell up to your left shoulder in an arc-motion to the Midpoint position. Pause briefly.

Lower left dumbbell back down in an arc-motion to Start/Finish position.

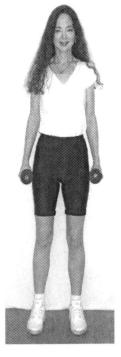   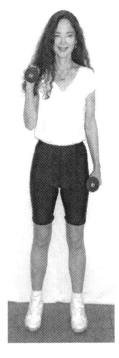

Start/Finish position   **Midpoint position**

Exercise 3: SHOULDERS--SIDE RAISE

Equipment: Dumbbell weights.

For each repetition:

Stand upright with feet about shoulder-width apart and abdominal muscles tightened. Avoid locking knees. Remember to keep breathing, don't hold your breath, and when possible exhale as you lift weights.

Start/Finish position: Hold dumbbells down in front of your thighs with palms facing inward toward outside of your thighs.

While keeping elbows slightly bent, extend and raise dumbbells out to your sides in arc-movements until they are level with your shoulders and your palms are facing down, which is the Midpoint position. Pause briefly.

While keeping arms nearly straight and palms facing down, lower dumbbells back to the sides of your thighs in arc-movements to the Start/Finish position.

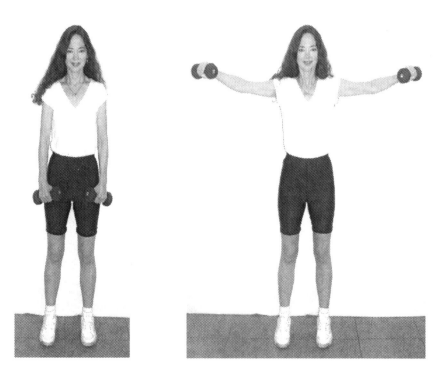

Start/Finish position   **Midpoint position**

Exercise 4: SHOULDERS--OVERHEAD PRESS

Equipment: Dumbbell weights.

For each repetition:

Stand upright with feet about shoulder-width apart and abdominal muscles tightened. Avoid locking knees. Remember to keep breathing, don't hold your breath, and when possible exhale as you lift weights.

<u>Start/Finish</u> position: Hold dumbbells just above shoulders with wrists facing forward and elbows lowered.

Press dumbbells straight up over shoulders keeping wrists facing forward to <u>Midpoint</u> position and continue to press. Pause briefly.

Lower dumbbells straight down to <u>Start/Finish</u> position.

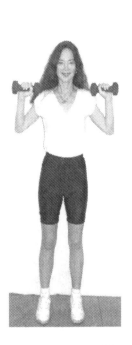

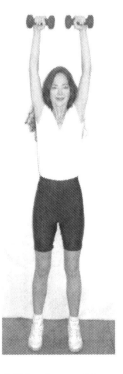

<u>Start/Finish</u> position   **<u>Midpoint</u> position**

Exercise 5: BACK--BENT LIFT

Equipment: Dumbbell weights.

For each repetition:

Stand with feet about shoulder-width apart. Bend forward at waist, look up and to the front, and keep your knees slightly bent. Your spine should be straight and your shoulders should not be rounded. Remember to keep breathing, don't hold your breath, and when possible exhale as you lift weights.

<u>Start/Finish</u> position: Hold dumbbells straight down in front of your legs with palms facing back toward your legs.

Keeping palms facing back, raise dumbbells straight up drawing your elbows up toward the ceiling in a rowing motion until the dumbbells are outside of and slightly lower than your shoulders to the <u>Midpoint</u> position. Squeeze shoulder blades together and pause briefly.

Keeping palms facing back, lower dumbbells back down to <u>Start/Finish</u> position.

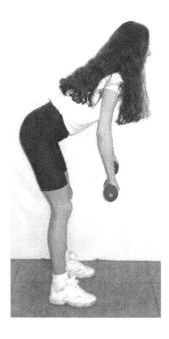 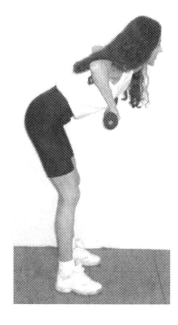

<u>Start/Finish</u> position　　　　　　**<u>Midpoint</u> position**

Exercise 6: BACK--UPRIGHT ROW

Equipment: Dumbbell weights.

For each repetition:

Stand up straight with feet about shoulder-width apart and abdominal muscles tightened. Avoid locking knees. Remember to keep breathing, don't hold your breath, and when possible exhale as you lift weights.

<u>Start/Finish</u> position: Hold dumbbells down in front of your legs with palms facing back toward your legs and with the inside ends of the dumbbells touching each other.

Raise dumbbells straight up along the front of your body to your chest with your elbows pointing out to the sides, palms facing your body, and the inside ends of dumbbells still touching each other to the <u>Midpoint</u> position. Pause briefly.

Keeping palms facing your body, lower dumbbells back down to <u>Start/Finish</u> position.

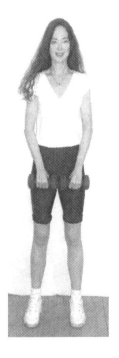   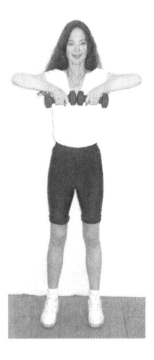

<u>**Start/Finish**</u> **position**   <u>**Midpoint**</u> **position**

Exercise 7: TRICEPS--EXTENSIONS

Equipment: Dumbbell weights.

For each repetition:

Stand with knees slightly bent (hips forward) and feet about shoulder-width apart or sit on bench with your back straight. Remember to keep breathing, don't hold your breath, and when possible exhale as you lift the weight.

<u>Start/Finish</u> position: Hold each end of a single dumbbell straight up over head with your wrists facing forward and your palms facing up.

While keeping your biceps close to your head and your upper arms straight up, bend elbows lowering the dumbbell behind your head in an arc-movement to the <u>Midpoint</u> position. Pause briefly.

Raise dumbbell back up in an arc-movement to the <u>Start/Finish</u> position.

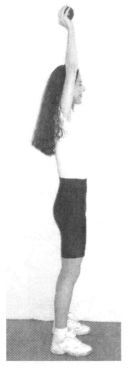   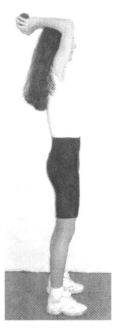

<u>Start/Finish</u> position   **<u>Midpoint</u> position**

Exercise 8: TRICEPS--PUSHBACK

Equipment: Dumbbell weights.

For each repetition:

Stand up straight with knees slightly bent. Look ahead and down slightly. Remember to keep breathing and when possible exhale as you lift weights.

<u>Start/Finish</u> position: Hold dumbbells close to the sides of your body near your hips with palms facing inward and with your upper arms and elbows pointing back.

While keeping your palms facing each other and your upper arms steady and elbows pointing back, extend your lower arms and dumbbells back in arc-movements until your arms are in the <u>Midpoint</u> position. Pause briefly.

Move dumbbells down and forward in arc-movements back to the <u>Start/Finish</u> position.

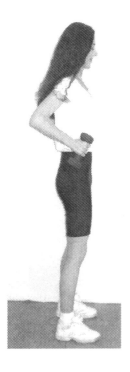

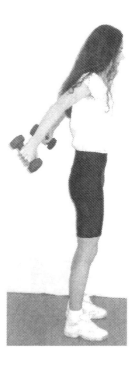

<u>Start/Finish</u> position   **<u>Midpoint</u> position**

Exercise 9: CHEST--FLYE

Equipment: Dumbbell weights and a bench or equivalent.

For each repetition:

Lie on your back on a bench. Remember to keep breathing, don't hold your breath, and when possible exhale as you lift weights.

<u>Start/Finish</u> position: Hold dumbbells straight up over your chest with your palms facing each other.

With elbows slightly bent, extend and lower dumbbells out to sides in arc-movements until they are just above chest level (out from your shoulders) at <u>Midpoint</u> position. Pause briefly.

While keeping elbows slightly bent but arms extended, raise dumbbells up in arc-movements toward top and center to <u>Start/Finish</u> position.

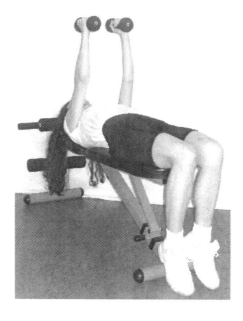
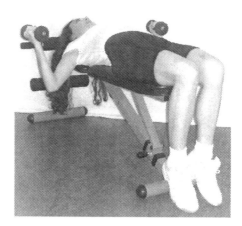

<u>Start/Finish</u> position   **<u>Midpoint</u> position**

Exercise 10: CHEST—BENCH PRESS

Equipment: Dumbbell weights and a bench or equivalent.

For each repetition:

Lie on your back on a bench. Remember to keep breathing, don't hold your breath, and when possible exhale as you lift weights.

Start/Finish position: Hold dumbbells down just above your shoulders with your palms facing up and elbows lowered.

Press dumbbells straight up over your chest to the Midpoint position and continue to press. Pause briefly.

Lower dumbbells to Start/Finish position.

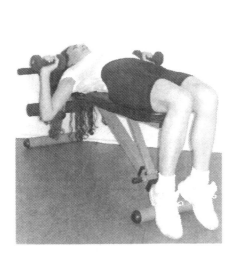
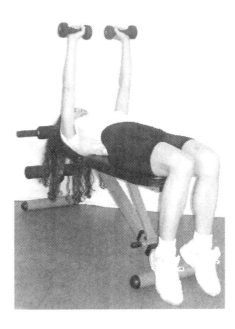

Start/Finish position   **Midpoint position**

LOWER-BODY EXERCISES

The following lower-body exercises are described in detail below. If possible, stand in front of a mirror to monitor your movements. Remember to use the *Cut-Out Pages of Daily Workout Summary* at the end of the book as a daily reference once you are more familiar with the exercises.

Exercise 1:   CALVES--STANDING STRAIGHT-TOE RAISE
Exercise 2:   CALVES--STANDING TOES ANGLED-OUT RAISE

Exercise 3:   QUADRICEPS/GLUT--SQUAT
Exercise 4:   QUADRICEPS/GLUT--SQUAT (Repeat Exercise 3)
Exercise 5:   QUADRICEPS--EXTENSION

Exercise 6:   HAMSTRING--CURLS
Exercise 7:   HAMSTRING--LUNGE

Exercise 8:   ABDOMINAL--LEG LOWERING
Exercise 9:   ABDOMINAL--CRUNCH
Exercise 10: ABDOMINAL--ALTERNATE TWIST

Note that you may use a weight bench with a built in leg-extension and leg-curl mechanism for doing Exercise 5: QUADRICEPS--EXTENSION and Exercise 6: HAMSTRING—CURLS.

Exercise 1: CALVES--STANDING STRAIGHT-TOE RAISE

Equipment: Dumbbell weights.

For each repetition:

Stand up straight with legs straight and feet about shoulder-width apart. Remember to keep breathing, don't hold your breath, and when possible exhale as you rise.

<u>Start/Finish</u> position: Point feet straight forward and hold a dumbbell in each hand down at your sides with palms facing inward toward the outside of your thighs.

While keeping your legs straight, raise up on your toes as far as possible to the <u>Midpoint</u> position.

Lower back down until your heels are touching the floor to the <u>Start/Finish</u> position.

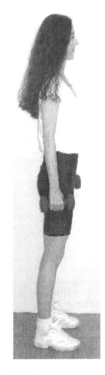   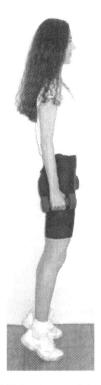

<u>Start/Finish</u> position   **<u>Midpoint</u> position**

Exercise 2: CALVES--STANDING TOES ANGLED-OUT RAISE

Equipment: Dumbbell weights.

For each repetition:

Stand up straight with legs straight and feet about shoulder-width apart. Remember to keep breathing, don't hold your breath, and when possible exhale as you rise.

<u>Start/Finish</u> position: Point feet out to sides about half way between straight forward and sideways and hold a dumbbell in each hand down at your sides with palms facing inward toward the outside of your thighs.

While keeping your legs straight, raise up on your toes as far as possible to the <u>Midpoint</u> position.

Lower back down until your heels are touching the floor to the <u>Start/Finish</u> position.

Note: Stretch your calf muscles after work out. (Described before exercises.)

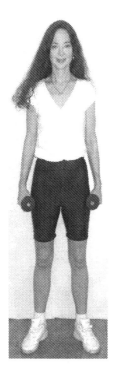

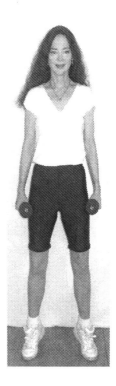

<u>Start/Finish</u> position   **<u>Midpoint</u> position**

Exercise 3: QUADRICEPS/GLUT--SQUAT

Equipment: Dumbbell weights.

For each repetition:

Stand up straight with feet about shoulder-width apart. Remember to keep breathing, don't hold your breath, and when possible exhale as you lower.

<u>Start/Finish</u> position: Point feet slightly outward and hold a dumbbell in each hand down at your sides with palms facing inward toward the outside of your thighs.

While keeping arms down at your sides and your back, head, and shoulders straight and nearly upright, bend knees and lower your hips until your upper legs are approaching parallel with the floor, as if you are going to sit in a chair, to the <u>Midpoint</u> position. Note: You may actually lower yourself and sit on the edge of a chair. Be careful not to lower yourself too far to avoid straining your knees.

Raise your body back up to <u>Start/Finish</u> position.

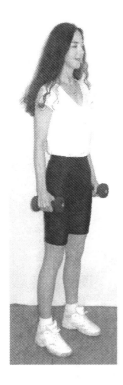   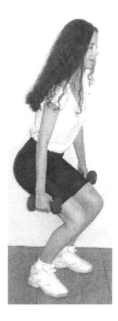

<u>**Start/Finish**</u> **position**   <u>**Midpoint**</u> **position**

Exercise 4: QUADRICEPS/GLUT--SQUAT (repeat of Exercise 3)

Exercise 5: QUADRICEPS--EXTENSION

Note: A weight bench with a leg extension mechanism may be used.

Equipment: Ankle weights (or a dumbbell weight) and a bench or equivalent.

For each repetition:

Sit on a bench with feet down and hold on to sides of bench. Remember to keep breathing, don't hold your breath, and when possible exhale as you lift legs.

<u>Start/Finish</u> position: Either strap ankle weights around each ankle or hold a dumbbell between your feet.

Keeping your body and upper legs stationary, extend your lower legs forward in an arc-motion until your knees are straight and your feet are in the <u>Midpoint</u> position. Pause briefly.

Lower your feet back down in an arc-motion to <u>Start/Finish</u> position.

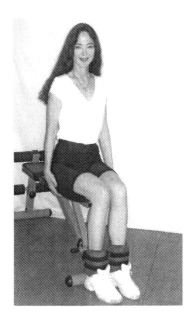

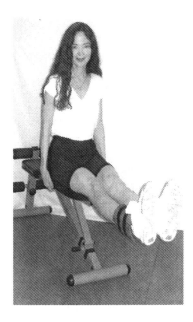

<u>Start/Finish</u> position   **<u>Midpoint</u> position**

Exercise 6: HAMSTRING--CURLS

Note: A weight bench with a hamstring curl mechanism may be used instead.

Equipment: Ankle weights. This exercise may be performed standing up holding onto a chair, or on a pad lying face down on the floor.

For each repetition:

Strap ankle weights onto each ankle and stand up while holding onto the back of a chair. Remember to keep breathing and when possible exhale as lower leg rises.

Start/Finish position: Standing up holding the back of a chair with ankle weights strapped to each ankle and legs straight.

Keeping your body and upper legs stationary, bend one knee raising lower leg and foot up in an arc-motion until your knee is at a 90-degree angle and your foot is in the Midpoint position. Pause briefly.

Lower foot back down in an arc-motion to Start/Finish position.

Repeat this exercise using the other leg.

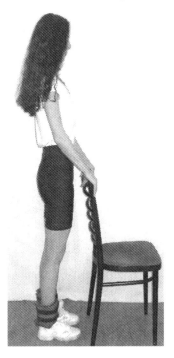 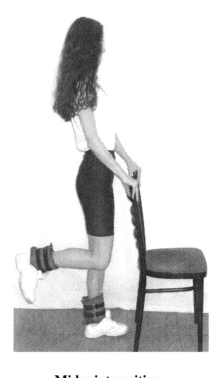

Start/Finish position   **Midpoint position**

(To perform this exercise lying down: lie face down on a pad with your arms crossed supporting your head and ankle weights strapped to each ankle. Start/Finish position: Lie face down with legs straight. Keeping your body and upper legs stationary, bend knees raising lower legs and feet up in an arc-motion until your feet are nearly up over your knees in Midpoint position. Pause briefly. Lower feet back down to Start/Finish position.)

Exercise 7: HAMSTRING--LUNGE

Equipment: Dumbbell weights.

For each repetition:

Stand up straight with feet about shoulder-width apart. Remember to keep breathing, don't hold your breath, and when possible exhale as you lower.

<u>Start/Finish</u> position: Point feet forward and hold a dumbbell in each hand down at your sides with palms facing inward toward the outside of your thighs.

While keeping arms down and your back, head, and shoulders straight and upright, step forward with your left foot bending your knees and lowering your hips until your right knee is several inches above the floor (or as close to the floor as you are comfortable) to the <u>Midpoint</u> position. The knee of your forward leg should not go past your forward foot.

Push with your forward leg, raising your body back up and step back to <u>Start/Finish</u> position.

Repeat by stepping forward with your right foot and lowering your left knee.

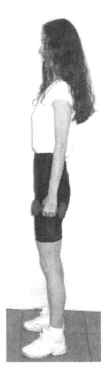 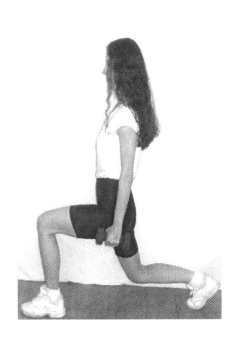

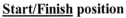

<u>Start/Finish</u> position   **<u>Midpoint</u> position**

Exercise 8: ABDOMINAL--LEG LOWERING

Equipment: None.

For each repetition:

Lie on your back on the floor or a pad with your arms down at your sides and hands slightly supporting your hips. Remember to keep breathing, don't hold your breath, and when possible exhale as legs lower.

<u>Start/Finish</u> position: Keeping the middle of your back touching the floor, hold your legs up in the air with your feet together and your knees slightly bent.

Keeping the middle of your back against the floor lower legs about 6 inches (away from your head) to the <u>Midpoint</u> position. Pause briefly.

Lift your legs back up to the <u>Start/Finish</u> position.

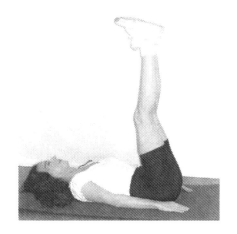
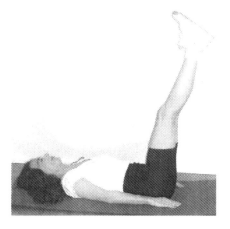

<u>Start/Finish</u> position   **<u>Midpoint</u> position**

Exercise 9: ABDOMINAL--CRUNCH

Equipment: None.

For each repetition:

Lie on your back on the floor or a pad with your knees bent and shoulder width apart and feet flat on the floor. Remember to keep breathing, don't hold your breath, and when possible exhale during lift.

<u>Start/Finish</u> position: Keeping your shoulders on the floor, lift your head so that your chin is close to touching your chest (you are looking toward your knees) and your arms are reaching toward your knees.

Keeping your chin to your chest (looking toward your knees), lift your shoulders up from the floor as your hands reach further between your knees to the <u>Midpoint</u> position. Pause briefly.

Lower your shoulders back down to the floor to the <u>Start/Finish</u> position, keeping your chin close to your chest.

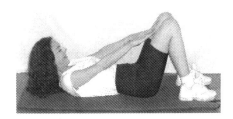   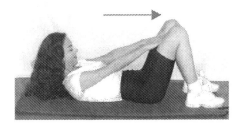

<u>Start/Finish</u> position   **<u>Midpoint</u> position**

Exercise 10: ABDOMINAL--ALTERNATE TWIST

Equipment: None.

For each repetition:

Lie on your back on the floor or a pad. Remember to keep breathing and when possible exhale as your elbow moves toward the opposite knee.

<u>Start</u> position: Hold your arms behind your head with fingers just touching your head behind your ears, knees bent and pointing up, and feet flat on the floor.

Point your right leg half way between straight up and the floor and raise your left knee back toward your right shoulder while pointing your right elbow toward your left knee. Your left elbow is on the floor. This is <u>Midpoint</u> position 1.

Switch the positions of your legs while rotating your shoulders so that your left leg is pointing half way between straight up and the floor, your right knee is pointing back toward your left shoulder, and your left elbow is pointing toward your right knee. Your right elbow is on the floor. This is <u>Midpoint</u> position 2. Switch back and forth by rotating shoulders and reversing leg positions to alternate between the two midpoint positions.

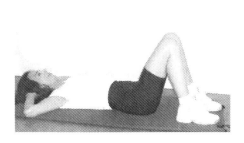

<u>Start</u> position

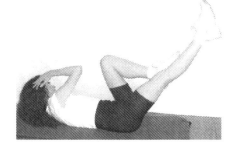

<u>Midpoint</u> position 1: Right leg out, left knee back, and left elbow on floor.

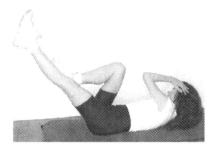

<u>Midpoint</u> position 2: Left leg out, right knee back, and right elbow on floor.

Chapter 5

Sleep Well

Don't turn to food for the energy you
should be getting from adequate sleep

"Would you like to go down to the cafeteria for an afternoon pick-me-up snack?" Ellen asked Isabelle as they approached each other in the hallway at work.

"I'm not hungry, but I'll join you and have some sparkling water," Isabelle replied.

"How do you go all afternoon without a snack? Don't you get tired?" Ellen asked as they headed for the cafeteria.

"I get eight hours of sleep every night—can't survive without it," Isabelle responded.

"How do you manage to get all that sleep? I'm lucky if I get six hours!" Ellen said.

"I used to get only six hours of sleep too—and also needed a daily afternoon pick-me-up snack. That was thirty pounds ago when I used to stay up late in front of the TV every night and eat," Isabelle smiled as she opened the door to the cafeteria.

"I was wondering how you lost all that weight—so how did you do it?" Ellen looked enviously at Isabelle's trim figure as they walked into the cafeteria.

"I got rid of my TV and stopped eating in the evening," Isabelle said as she reached for her sparkling water. *"That left more time for me to think and dream about my life and future."*

One hundred years ago, adults in the United States slept an average of 9 hours per night. Today, that average is less than 7 hours.[58] Since the mid-1960's, not only has the rate of obesity nearly tripled in the U.S., but there has been an average reduction of two hours from our nightly sleep. Some researchers believe there is a connection between sleep and body weight, and it may be due to sleep's effect on the blood concentrations of hunger and satiety hormones, which affect eating behavior.[59] When we don't get adequate and healthy sleep, we become tired and feel hungry even though our bodies don't need the calories. We also eat when we are not truly hungry because we need energy. Being tired because you haven't made adequate sleep a priority will cause you to eat more than you need "just to get through the day". Eating for the energy you should be getting from sleep is a mistake, and can sabotage your weight-control efforts. A top priority should be soundly sleeping 7 to 8 hours every night.

Sleep problems can exacerbate weight problems. People who don't get enough sleep due to their schedule or sleep disorders drag themselves around during the day and burn fewer calories. If their fatigue is due to sleep apnea and they gain weight, it actually worsens the apnea.[60] Sleep-deprived people may also make poor food choices and eat sugary foods to give themselves a momentary lift. They are less likely to have the energy to exercise. Preliminary studies also suggest a direct connection between inadequate sleep and insulin resistance, diabetes, cardiovascular disease, low-grade inflammation, and hormonal changes that promote weight gain.[61] Along with diet and exercise, healthy sleep provides the essential foundation for mental

---

[58] Science News v.160, No.2 Pg.31, 7/14/01

[59] Science News v.167, No.14 Pg.216, 5/2/05

[60] The Promise of Sleep, William C. Dement, M.D., Ph.D., Delacorte Press 1999 p.428

[61] Science News v.162 No.10, p.152-154, 9/7/02

and physical well-being. People who get adequate sleep tend to be more engaged and are better able to think through new ideas and carry more ideas in their head.[62]

Our weight and lifestyle affects our children, which is evidenced by the primary risk factor for childhood obesity being parental obesity. Other significant risk factors for childhood obesity include low parental concern regarding the child's weight and the child having a sensitive disposition. It also is significant that on average overweight children obtain 30 fewer minutes of sleep than normal-weight children.[63] In general, while individuals can vary, it is accepted that adults need approximately 7 to 8 hours of sleep in a 24-hour period, children and teenagers require more sleep, and older adults may require slightly less.

What Is Sleep?

There are key indicators of sleep that are demonstrated by most mammals. These indicators include muscle relaxation, changes in brain-wave activity, changes in body temperature, the presence of *rapid eye movement* sleep and its characteristic brain-wave patterns, and the perceptual disengagement of the brain from sensory stimulation in the environment. There are various stages of sleep, each with its characteristic electrical brain wave patterns.[64] Sleep is often divided into two primary types based on patterns of brain electrical activity measured with an electroencephalogram (EEG), as well as on eye movements and muscle tone. These two types are called *rapid eye movement* (REM) sleep or *paradoxical sleep* and *non-rapid eye movement* sleep (non-REM) or *slow wave sleep. Rapid eye movement* sleep is identified by rapid eye movements, decreased muscular tone, and low-amplitude fast rhythms on electro-encephalographic recordings. *Slow wave sleep* or *non-rapid eye movement* sleep is characterized by large-amplitude, low-frequency electroencephalographic oscillations. The REM/non-REM cycle in humans typically has a 90-min period.[65]

The *function of sleep* is not well understood, although researchers are increasing their understanding of the processes involved in generating and maintaining sleep. Researchers speculate that these processes include energy

---

[62] The Promise of Sleep, William C. Dement, M.D., Ph.D., Delacorte Press 1999 p.312

[63] Stanford Report, July 21, 2004

[64] The Promise of Sleep, William C. Dement, M.D., Ph.D. , Delacorte Press 1999 p.17,18,241,248

[65] Science v.294, p.1048-1052, 11/2/01; Science v.294, p.1052-1057, 11/2/01

conservation, brain thermoregulation, brain detoxification, tissue restoration, and brain plasticity relating to learning and memory.[66] When we are asleep, biochemical processes occur that are important for the healthy functioning of our bodies. During sleep, sugars are stored, the body temperature decreases which conserves energy, various hormones and chemicals including prolactin, cortisol, and growth hormone (which promotes tissue repair) are released into the bloodstream, and the immune system is boosted with the increase in levels of immune system chemicals such as interleukin-1 and tumor necrosis factor (which is a killer of cancer cells) in the blood.[67] In fact, a study suggested that sleep not only affects natural immunity, but even modest disturbances of sleep reduce natural killer cell activity in humans.[68]

During the REM stage of sleep when we *dream* the brain is very active. Researchers believe there is a connection between sleep and memory, with some research suggesting that memories may be processed during REM sleep.[69] Research involving genetics, neurophysiology, and the neurosciences provides evidence that supports a role for sleep in learning, memory tasks, and the reprocessing of memories.[70] There are also research findings that non-REM, or slow wave, sleep may play a role in learning.[71] The consolidation of different types of memory seems to be tied to different sleep stages.[72] While researchers do not agree on the specific role of sleep in memory consolidation, most experts agree that sleep is important for learning and performing tasks.[73] There is growing research and evidence supporting the role of sleep in memory processing and consolidation after learning or training. Sleep has been shown to increase overnight learning on memory tasks.[74] Even learning procedural skills in which performance improves significantly with practice, improvement on tasks continues in the absence of further practice during periods of sleep and not across equivalent waking periods. Sleep-dependent procedural skill learning has been demonstrated across various skill domains, including visual, auditory, and motor.[75]

---

[66] Science v.294, p.1048-1052, 11/2/01

[67] The Promise of Sleep, William C. Dement, M.D., Ph.D. , Delacorte Press 1999 p.258,266,268

[68] Psychosomatic Medicine v. 56, Issue 6 493-498, 1994

[69] August 2000 Nature Neuroscience/in Science v.289, No..5479, p539, 7/28/00; Science News v.158, No.4, p.55, 7/22/00

[70] Science v.294, p.1052, 11/2/01; Science v.294, p.1048, 11/2/01; Science v.294, p.1052, 11/2/01

[71] Science News v.161, No.22, p.341, 6/1/02

[72] Born and Gais 2003, Roles of Early and Late Nocturnal Sleep for the Consolidation of Human Memories
In Sleep and Brain Plasticity, eds Maquet et al. p65-85, Oxford University Press, New York

[73] Science v..294, p.1058-1063, 11/2/01

[74] Neuroscience v.133, p.911-917, 2005

[75] Cerebral Cortex v.15 No.11 p.1666, 2005; Nat. Neurosci. v.3, p.1335, 2000; Nat. Neurosci. v.3, p.1237, 2000; J. Cogn. Neurosci.
v.12, p246, 2000; J. Cogn.Neurosci. v.16, p.53, 2004; Neuroreport v.15, p.731, 2004; Proc.Natl.Acad.Sci v.99, p.11987, 2002;
Neuron v.35, p.205, 2002; Nature v.425, p.516, 2003; Learn.Mem. v10, p.275, 2003; Proc.Natl.Acad.Sci. v.100, p.12492, 2003;
J.Exp. Psychol. Hum. Precept. Perform. v.9, p.86, 2004

In fact, *sleep deprivation* has been shown to impair subsequent performance on various tasks in both animals and humans.[76] Research also suggests that sleep in early life may play a crucial role in brain development.[77] In particular, both REM and non-REM sleep may be important to brain development. While REM sleep has long been thought to be important for the development of neurons in the young brain, non-REM sleep may also play a role in brain development.[78]

We have much to learn about the precise roles of sleep in brain development, learning, memory, and the functioning of our bodies and immune systems. What we do know is that sleep is extremely important and should not be neglected.

Sleep Deprivation

When our lives become busy, sleep is usually one of the first areas where we sacrifice. When we are sleep deprived, our cognitive functions are adversely affected. After a sleepless night, brain functions measured during certain types of thought actually change. It was revealed in a study that sleep-deprived adults were shown to exhibit an unusual pattern of brain activity as they attempted to memorize words, and also displayed lower brain activity while trying to solve math problems.[79] In another study, participants tried to memorize short lists of words the day after a full night of sleep, and then after 35 hours without sleep. Word recall and recognition dropped sharply after sleep deprivation.[80] In yet another study, participants performed various arithmetic tasks involving subtraction. These participants made more mistakes and omitted more responses when sleepy.[81]

Another link between the brain and sleep was demonstrated in a study of rats, which found that rats deprived of sleep for 72 hours had higher levels of the stress hormone corticosterone, and produced significantly fewer new brain cells in a particular region of the hippocampus (a part of the brain involved in learning and memory).[82]

---

[76] Science v.294, p.1048-1052, 11/2/01

[77] Neuron v.30, No1, p.275, Apr 2001

[78] Nature Reviews Neuroscience v.2, p.383, 2001

[79] Science News v.157, No.71, p.103, 2/12/00

[80] Nature 2/10/2000 /Science News v.157, No.71, p.103, 2/12/00

[81] NeuroReport 12/16/99 /Science News v.157, No.71, p.103, 2/12/00

[82] Proceedings of the National Academy of Science v.103, No.50, p.19170, 12/12/06

Studies that have examined resident-physicians' moods and attitudes have also demonstrated deleterious effects of sleep deprivation and fatigue. It has been shown that while sleep deprived or fatigued residents can compensate for sleep loss in crises or other novel situations, these sleep-deprived residents may be more prone to errors on routine, repetitive tasks, and tasks that require sustained vigilance, which comprise a substantial portion of a resident's workload.[83]

Prolonged and severe sleep deprivation is also associated with alterations of natural and cellular immune function. Even a modest disturbance of sleep or just partial night's sleep deprivation has been shown to reduce natural immune system responses in humans.[84]

When and how well we sleep determines our sleep/wake cycle (circadian rhythm) and can alter the balance of hormones in our bodies. Because of its effect on hormones, the sleep/wake cycle is a possible link to a person's cancer risk. Hormones affected by sleep include melatonin, estrogen, and cortisol. When the circadian rhythm is disrupted, the body produces less melatonin, which is involved in removing damaging free-radical compounds, and therefore its suppression may allow the cell's DNA to be more susceptible to cancer-causing mutations. Melatonin also may be useful against cancer because it slows the ovaries' production of estrogen, and for many ovarian and breast tumors, the presence of estrogen stimulates the cancerous cells to continue dividing. There is also a possible link between breast cancer and cortisol, and people whose cortisol cycle is shifted by troubled sleep may be more susceptible to cancer. Night-shift workers have been shown to have a higher rate of breast cancer than women who sleep normal hours.[85]

It is important to get enough sleep for other more immediate reasons. Even a few nights with little or no sleep can cause someone to become a danger to himself or others. People suffering from insomnia and sleep disorders that prevent them from obtaining adequate sleep are more likely to have automobile accidents and other serious accidents. In fact, 33 percent of traffic accidents can be traced to sleepiness, and in a Gallup Poll, 31 percent of respondents said they have dozed off at the wheel of an automobile.[86]

---

[83] Academic Medicine v.66, p.687, 1991

[84] The FASEB Journal v.10, p.643, 1996 by The Federation of American Societies for Experimental Biology

[85] Stanford Report, October 8, 2003, Psychiatric research builds link between sleep, stress, cancer progression

[86] The Promise of Sleep, William C. Dement, M.D., Ph.D., Delacorte Press 1999 p.137,225

If you can't get enough sleep at night (or during your normal sleep time), then consider napping.

Sleep Disorders

The most common symptom of a sleep disorder is daytime fatigue, which often manifests itself in lack of motivation, apathy, irritability, or feeling exhausted, depressed, or generally unhealthy. *Sleep disorders* can last days, weeks, or years, and may be caused by physical or mental illness, injury, toxicity, or demands of life that prevent us from staying on a regular sleep schedule. Types of sleep disorders include insomnia, sleep apnea, snoring, narcolepsy, restless legs syndrome, problems with the biological clock, REM sleep disorder, sleepwalking, and night terrors. The primary danger with sleep disorders is fatigue-induced accidents, and for sleep apnea, the danger of fatal arrhythmias, heart attacks, and strokes.[87]

A growing number of studies have linked *snoring* to heart disease and stroke. Snoring is more of a problem for people who are overweight and sleep-deprived. Both obesity and fatigue exacerbate snoring. Snoring is an indication that airflow is restricted. According to researchers, people who are snoring are struggling so hard to breathe that they are putting stress on their hearts.[88] Some researchers believe that people who do not correct their snoring will develop sleep apnea as they age, especially if they gain weight.[89]

Severe or loud snoring is linked to obstructive *sleep apnea*, in which loud snoring is frequently interrupted by episodes of stopped breathing. The severity of the disorder varies from having the airway close or collapse for seconds to minutes, to a partial closing of the airway called hypopnea, in which the sleeper gets less than a full breath. During as much as half of their sleep time, people with sleep apnea can have lower oxygen concentrations in their blood. This lack of oxygen causes the heart to pump harder to circulate blood faster, and over time can lead to irregular heartbeats or high blood pressure.[90] A person with sleep apnea stops breathing for up to 60 seconds or even longer, which can occur hundreds of times per night. This happens as

---

[87] The Promise of Sleep, William C. Dement, M.D., Ph.D., Delacorte Press 1999 p.128,345

[88] Science News v.157, No.11, p.172, 3/11/00; Robert Clark of Regional Sleep Disorders Center at Columbus Community Hosp.

[89] Regina Walker of Loyola University Medical Center, Science News v.157, No.11, p.172, 3/11/00

[90] Science News v.157, No.11, p.172, 3/11/00

soft tissues in the throat close, causing the diaphragm to struggle, while carbon dioxide builds up in the blood and oxygen drops dramatically depriving the brain and body. The victim awakes enough to gasp for breath, then falls asleep, repeating the cycle throughout the night, but not remembering any of it the next day. During the actual apnea, the heartbeat can slow nearly to a stop. When the apnea victim begins to breathe, oxygen levels rise again, but the heart starts pumping rapidly and blood pressure rises to a very high level. Over time this can damage organs and cause small strokes in the brain. The primary dangers connected with sleep apnea are its association with heart problems, high blood pressure, strokes, and the drowsiness that can cause accidents.

Sleep apnea is very often associated with obesity.[91] A recent large study found a link between sleep apnea with both glucose intolerance and impaired insulin function, which are associated with the onset of Type II diabetes.[92] There are additional risk factors for sleep apnea, which include not only fluctuations in blood pressure and heart rate, cardiovascular problems, and fragmented sleep, but also increased sympathetic activity, cortical arousal, and cognitive and behavioral problems.[93] In addition, untreated obstructive sleep apnea predisposes individuals to an increased risk of hypertension, and in support of this, treatment of obstructive sleep apnea lowers blood pressure, even during the daytime.[94]

Patients with obstructive sleep apnea often complain of daily forgetfulness including losing keys, forgetting phone numbers, or forgetting to complete daily tasks. A recent study[95] showed that the majority of patients with obstructive sleep apnea, who were memory-impaired prior to treatment with a continuous positive airway pressure (CPAP) machine, which was developed for treating sleep apnea, brought their memory up to normal memory performance after 3 months of using the CPAP machine at least 6 hours per night. The study also showed that memory improvement correlated positively with the number of hours the CPAP machine was used per night.

There are several treatments that have been developed for sleep apnea including a continuous positive airway pressure (CPAP) machine, a radio frequency technology procedure, *weight loss*, nasal continuous positive

---

[91] The Promise of Sleep, William C. Dement, M.D., Ph.D., Delacorte Press 1999 p.168,178,177,174,181

[92] Science News v.166, No.13, p.195, 9/25/04

[93] JAMA v.291, p2013, 4/28/04

[94] Hypertension. v.42, p.1067, 11/10/03

[95] CHEST v.130 p.1772, Dec. 2006

airway pressure (N-CPAP), pharyngeal surgery, and medications.[96] The one non-invasive potentially curative treatment is weight loss.

While obstructive sleep apnea syndrome is a well-recognized cause of excessive sleepiness, *mild* sleep-disordered breathing may also be related to sleepiness. It is believed to affect as much as half the adult population. It was found that sleep-disordered breathing is associated with excess sleepiness in a group of middle-aged and older adults, and was not limited to those with clinically apparent sleep apnea.[97] Anyone who snores regularly, pauses in breathing while asleep, is sleepy during the day, experiences a dry throat in the morning, has night sweats, has morning headaches, is overweight, or has unexplained hypertension should consult a physician.[98]

Other sleep disorders include *insomnias,* which can be caused by stress, worry, jet lag, schedule changes, a noisy sleep environment, biological rhythm problems, or schedules that conflict with a person's natural awake-sleep times. Persistent insomnias can also be linked to *restless legs syndrome*, *gastroesophageal reflux*, and *fibromyalgia.*

Inadequate or poor sleep can cause you to be unnecessarily unhealthy because most sleep problems are treatable.

---

[96] Crit Rev Oral Biol Med, v.15, No.3, p.137, 2004; American Journal of Respiratory and Critical Care Medicine v.159, No.6, p.1884, June 1999; Chest, v.109, p.1346, 1996, American College of Chest Physicians; The Promise of Sleep, Dement, M.D., Ph.D., Delacorte Press 1999 p.181,186-90

[97] American Journal of Respiratory and Critical Care Medicine, v.159, No.2, p.502, February 1999

[98] Science News v.157, No.11, p.172, 3/11/00

Tips on Improving Sleep and Getting to Sleep

Generally accepted recommendations on improving and getting to sleep include the following:

1. Avoid caffeine (in coffee, black tea, or soft drinks), particularly in the late afternoon and evening;
2. Eat dinner at least 3 hours before bedtime (not a problem on *3:00 PM days*!);
3. Maintain a regular bedtime schedule;
4. Relax before going to bed (reading is recommended);
5. Keep your bedroom quiet throughout the night or use white noise such as a fan or air cleaner;
6. Maintain your room at a comfortable temperature;
7. Keep the bedroom dark and use dim nightlights to avoid turning on bright lights during your sleep time; and
8. Exercise regularly (although not right before bedtime).

Many people stay up watching television programs out of habit, not because they are interesting or beneficial. Turn off the television and stop other activities 9 hours before you have to get up. Then you will have an hour to get ready for the next day and for bed. In fact, researchers believe there is a potential negative impact from television viewing at bedtime for children. In particular, the presence of a television set in a child's bedroom may be a contributor to sleep problems in school children.[99] I suspect this holds true for adults as well.

Finally, don't sabotage your weight-control efforts by eating to 'keep going' because you are tired or sleepy. The cure is simply more quality sleep.

---

[99] PEDIATRICS v.104, No.3, p.e27, September 1999

Chapter 6

Successful Aging

Madeline is older than Isabelle, and they are both excellent word processors and typists. Isabelle noticed how fast Madeline typed and challenged her to a race to see who was faster. Madeline figured she would win because she has decades more experience than her young friend. Isabelle was certain she would win because she is younger and faster. The race was on—and it was a tie! While the speed of each individual keystroke was slower for Madeline, she could type just as fast as Isabelle by reading further ahead and more efficiently anticipating the next key. To celebrate their co-victory, they went out for a late lunch. Madeline was fascinated with Isabelle's description of Tahiti – and how she got there. After listening to her younger friend excitedly extol the virtues of her new lifestyle and dreams, Madeline decided to adopt The 3:00 PM Secret for herself and began looking forward to a long and vital life full of new adventures in a new, fit body.

To Isabelle's surprise, older typists were found to type just as fast as younger typists by reading ahead and anticipating the next key, even though the speed of each individual keystroke was slower.[100] Although a person may slow down the speed at which she performs certain skills, she can still accomplish any task–perhaps just a little bit more slowly. Any slowing that may occur as we age can be compensated for by the wisdom and experience that we have gained over our lifetimes. When it comes to thinking and making decisions, the results are even better. The speed at which we make decisions may slow somewhat with age; nevertheless, applying wisdom and experience will result in better decisions!   Active, stimulated brains do not lose mental abilities that cannot be compensated for easily.

Good News on Aging

Many of the world's most productive and creative people are, and have been, older adults who make great contributions well into old age. Aging gives us the opportunity to learn, explore, and pursue our passions. By using what we are learning about nutrition, exercise, mental stimulation, stress, mindset, sleep, healthful living, hormones, and genetics, it is possible to push back disease and the aging process, extend our lives, and give ourselves more time to pursue our dreams. If treated properly, our bodies and brains do not need to decline nearly as much as we think they will, and the limited losses can be, and often are, compensated for by experience and wisdom. There are also many benefits to growing older. Included among these benefits are that older people are generally happier than younger people, have better social wisdom, possess the ability to more accurately evaluate a stranger's personality, and have better verbal abilities.[101]

I have included this chapter on *Successful Aging* in a book on weight control because I believe that many of the behaviors we apply to keeping our bodies healthy, slim, and fit, will also help us live longer, more vigorous, and happier lives. Practicing good habits in nutrition, exercise, sleep, stress-reduction, and positive mental stimulation during our 30's, 40's, 50's, 60's,

---

[100] Stealing Time: The New Science of Aging, Warshofsky, TV Books 1999 p.17,187,193

[101] Science v.299, No.5611, p.1300, 2/28/03

70's, 80's, and beyond, will promote a longer life in a strong, fit body. In addition, if I am helping and encouraging you to take care of your body so it lasts, it is only fair to consider how to make those extra years – or decades – worth sticking around to enjoy.

The question researchers have been trying to understand is why some people seem to decline mentally and physically while others remain strong in body and mind. Clearly, diseases can affect people's minds and bodies, but in the absence of Alzheimer's and related diseases or extreme physical illness or disability, there is still a great variation in mental and physical ability for people in their seventies and beyond. There are many factors that have been found to contribute to successful aging. A summary of characteristics found in various studies of people who age successfully includes higher levels of education and continual intellectual challenge (novelty) all through life, good nutritional habits, avoiding cardiovascular disease and other life-threatening diseases, avoiding too much stress exposure, higher levels of exercise and physical activity, good lung function, better socioeconomic status and occupation, positive emotions, more adaptive coping skills, maintaining a feeling of control over one's life, being religious, and being mentally tough.[102]

While lifespan is influenced by our genes, it is believed that genes affect longevity because of their impact on our physiological capacity throughout life, and that aging is not a preprogrammed process governed directly and completely by our genes.[103] This suggests that attention to lifestyle plays a significant role in aging.

The mental decline once thought to be inevitable in aging people actually does not occur for most healthy, active adults. A longitudinal study that began in 1956, called the Seattle Longitudinal Study of Aging,[104] has been evaluating how a range of core mental skills hold up as we age. The participants perform a series of tests for cognitive skills every seven years. The cognitive tests taken by the participants include arithmetic skills, vocabulary skills, proficiency with spatial orientation, and the ability to recognize patterns referred to as inductive reasoning. This study was designed to understand why some people remain bright and sharp and lead

---

[102] Stealing Time: The New Science of Aging, Warshofsky, TV Books 1999 p.180,195,205,224-32; Science News v.159,No.2, p324, 5/26/01

[103] Nature v.408, No.6809, p.268, 11/9/00

[104] Stealing Time: The New Science of Aging, Warshofsky, TV Books 1999 p.188-193/Schaie, K.W. Intellectual development in adulthood: The Seattle Longitudinal Study. New York: Cambridge University Press, 1996

exciting lives, while others become feeble and mentally deteriorate as they age.

When this study began, it was widely believed that people begin a steady decline mentally in their twenties and continue to decline throughout the remainder of their lives. Contrary to the conventional wisdom, the results have shown that for healthy people, there are no significant declines in their abilities well into the sixties and seventies, after which the results become variable. The results show that sixty-year-olds are scoring as well on cognitive tests as they did in their twenties. In fact, some skills don't even reach their peak until people reached their thirties and forties! There are some individuals who show some decline in cognitive skills between the sixties and eighties, and others who do not show much decline until the eighties. In the eighties, most people show some decline, but again, the decline varies and appears to depend on what skills the individual practices and maintains during his or her life. *Skills used don't decline, whereas skills not used are more likely to show some decline.* (Seems to me this is true at any age.) This study found that the people who don't decline and whose skills are maintained into later life have important characteristics in common. These include higher education and maintenance of intellectual skills (have a complex and intellectually stimulating environment), middle-class lifestyle, good health (absence of chronic diseases), high intellectual status of spouse, and a flexible approach to life. Perhaps the "flexible" people can more easily adapt to changes in their lives and in the world, and make lifestyle changes that are beneficial.

Research on centenarians[105] has found that most people who live to be 100 or older are ill only in the last few years of life and live independently well into their 90's. In this study, factors that seem to determine why some people function better than others at very old ages include what they eat, how much they exercise, their social networks, and how well they handle stress. Researchers also believe that as we use and stimulate our brains, we make and strengthen connections between nerve cells. Therefore, as age presents our brains with various assaults on nerve tissue, the more connections we have produced through using our brains will allow them to hold up better against the assaults.

---

[105] Science News v.159, No.10, p.156, 3/10/01

The Brain

Scientists once thought that mental decline with age is inevitable. With some exceptions, however, there is evidence that this is not the case at all. Throughout our lives and into old age, we do in fact make new connections in our brains from one neuron to another as we learn and put ourselves into stimulating environments. Neurons grow by making new branches, called *dendrites*, which are extensions of the neuron. Dendrites form a dense web of interconnecting cells that make contact with each other across *synapses*. These highly branched structures formed by dendrites process the signals that are generated at the thousands of synapses. Dendrites respond to signals by strengthening or weakening communication across the synapses. Repeated signals to a particular synapse may strengthen it, whereas other activity patterns may weaken a synapse's future responses. These changes are believed to be a key factor in learning and memory.[106]

It had been believed that neurons could not regrow or regenerate themselves in the event of damage after brain development ended. In fact, it had been believed that the brains of adult mammals do not generate any new nerve cells. In reality, neurons do develop in the adult mammalian brain, including in the hippocampus area of the brain. Newly developed neurons may be associated with memory formation.[107] There is much research and growing evidence that neurogenesis, which is the production of new neurons, occurs in certain areas of the adult brain of various animals including birds, mice, and primates. Recent evidence suggests that neurogenesis can occur in the neocortex, which is the brain region most concerned with higher brain functions, such as learning and memory. The implications of these findings include the potential development of treatments that would stimulate neurogenesis in people who have, for example, Alzheimer's disease or spinal cord injury.[108] The discovery that neural stem cells exist throughout life in the adult brain and can renew and give rise to new neurons, astrocytes, and oligodendrocytes, just as occurs in the developing brain, revealed that neurogenesis can occur, and there is no requirement for a complex neuron to divide in order to create a new one. It is now known that neurons can be generated from primitive cells, similar to what happens in development.[109]

---

[106] Science v.290, No.5492 p.736, 10/27/00

[107] Nature v.410, No.6826, p.314, 372, 3/15/01

[108] Science v.288, No.5474, p.2111, 6/23/00; Nature v.407, p.963, 10/26/00; Science v.290, No.5492 p.735, 10/27/00

[109] The Journal of Neuroscience, v.22, No.3, p.612, 2/1/02

Various research studies have shown that neurogenesis occurs in the human brain and that the adult nervous system can generate new neurons.[110]

There is evidence that our activities can affect new growth in our brains. In studies on rats, researchers found that rats that grew up in a complex environment had an enlarged vascular system in their brains allowing more blood supply. In addition, if rats (including older rats) were placed into a stimulating environment, major changes occurred in their brains within a few days. These changes included many new dendrites forming many new synaptic connections, and also new blood vessels were formed thereby increasing the blood supply in their brains. These studies also demonstrated that *exercise* primarily stimulated an increase in *vasculature* and *blood flow* in their brains, whereas *learning* new tasks primarily stimulated growth of new *dendrites* and *synaptic connections* in their brains.[111] If we extrapolate to humans, this work suggests that if we learn new things, we will grow new dendrites and synaptic connections in our brains, and if we exercise, we will increase the vasculature and blood flow in our brains. Both are important.

It has been shown that if we stop using our brains at any age, our dendrites can retract and affect us cognitively. This is similar to a muscle getting smaller if you stop using it. Retracting dendrites can cause a loss in computational power, which is why *continuing to learn and stimulate our brains is so important at any age.* The good news is that dendrites can grow at any age as we use our brains and learn. In fact, it has been shown that learning alters the structure and function of the brain, and that changes occurring in synapses (the connections between neurons) are associated with different types of learning.[112] Researchers have also shown that intense learning and the acquisition of a great amount of highly abstract information appears to be related to a particular pattern of structural gray matter changes in specific brain areas, showing a significant increase in gray matter.[113]

The reason I cite these studies on brain research (and there are numerous similar studies I could include) is to communicate that the brain is dynamic and we can improve it and keep it acting young, or we can neglect it and let it deteriorate. Just like our muscles we can strengthen brain connections and

---

[110] Science (Adv. online pub.) DOI: 10.1126/science.1136281, 2/15/07; Annual Review of Neuroscience, v.28, p.223, July 2005; Annual Review of Pharmacology and Toxicology, v.44, p.399, February 2004

[111] Beckman News-Summer/Fall 1996 (V. 6/No. 2)/ http://www.beckman.uiuc.edu/outreach/bnfeature96.html; Proceedings of the National Academy of Sciences, v.87, p.5568-5572

[112] Curr Opin Neurobiol. v.9, No.2, p.203, Apr.1999 /Science v.289, No.5478, p.399, 7/21/00

[113] The Journal of Neuroscience, v.26,No.23,p.6314, 6/7/06

computational power with use or let our brains and bodies deteriorate with disuse. The fact that it is possible to keep our brains fully functional well into old age should provide even more motivation to keep our bodies in tip-top shape.

Factors that Affect Aging and Lifespan

Scientists have extended the *lifespans* of many different animals in laboratories. During the extended old-age period, the animals were healthy and vital, and appeared younger than their chronological ages. The implications of current animal research are that human lifespans may be increased to 150 to 200 years in the future. Living creatures are sometimes thought of as *self-repairing* beings who have mechanisms to heal wounds, mend bone tissue, and recover from disease, injury, and other assaults on the body. Many biologists think our aging is determined in a large part by our capacity for continual self-repair.

What factors contribute to helping our bodies stay healthy longer? Research is in progress on a number of factors that allow animals to have an increased lifespan in a body that remains younger than its chronological age. A number of factors that are known to affect the *aging process* and *lifespan* include: education and continued learning, exercise, stress, antioxidants and vitamins, calorie restriction, and avoidance of Alzheimer's disease. Making positive changes in lifestyle along with obtaining appropriate medical intervention later in life can notably improve your life expectancy.[114] Our lifespans can be increased by changes made later in life.

Education and Aging

One of the best activities for our brains is to stimulate them by learning and exposing ourselves to new ideas, new information, challenges, and novelty. Researchers have found that the connections between nerve cells (synapses) of more highly educated people were much denser than those of less educated people. This may allow healthy regions of the brain to take over for parts of the brain that have been damaged by Alzheimer's and similar diseases.[115] In an epidemiological study in Shanghai, China, over 5,000

---

[114] Science v.301, No.5640, p.1679, 9/19/03

[115] Stealing Time: The New Science of Aging, Fred Warshofsky, TV Books 1999 p.205; Odyssey—The Magazine of University of Kentucky Research, Summer/Fall 1994

people were followed for a decade, and more than a quarter of these people did not attend school when they were children. The non-educated individuals were found to be at a much greater risk of developing Alzheimer's disease and other dementing illnesses than those who attended school.[116]

A brain scan study of older adults showed that those with more education seem to be less affected cognitively by the brain shrinkage that accompanies aging. Researchers believe that mental activity creates a richer and more redundant array of connections between nerve cells in the brain, and that stronger connections are better able to resist small insults to the brain. This research is consistent with numerous other studies that demonstrate people with more *education* live longer and postpone the onset of dementia.[117]

The development of Alzheimer's disease later in life appears to be affected by environmental factors operating over the course of a lifetime. Research in North America, Europe, Asia, and the Middle East has shown that the incidence and prevalence of Alzheimer's disease is lower in people with relatively higher levels of education.[118] According to one study, each year of education in a person's life reduced the risk of Alzheimer's disease by 17%.[119] It has also been found that bilingualism has a protective effect in delaying the onset of dementia by an average of four years.[120]

Certain mental exercises were shown to counteract expected declines in the cognitive skills of 2,802 healthy independently living adults age 65 and older.[121] Participants in the study were divided into four groups, three of which took part in 10 training sessions targeting a specific cognitive ability—memory, reasoning, or speed of processing. The fourth group received no cognitive training. Sixty percent of those who completed the initial training took part in booster sessions designed to maintain improvements gained from the initial sessions. Immediately after the initial training, 87 percent of the speed-training group, 74 percent of the reasoning group, and 26 percent of the memory group showed improvement in the skills taught. After five years, people in each group performed better on tests in their respective areas of training than did people in the control group. This study showed that seniors

---

[116] Archives of Neurology v.51, p1220, 1994; http://medicine.ucsd.edu/neurosci/the-faculty/katzman.html

[117] Science v. 285, No. 5428, p 661, 7/30/99

[118] Neurology v.43, p.13, 1993; Ann. Neurol. v.27, p.428, 1990; Arch. Neurol. (Chicago) v.54, p.1399, 1997; Arch. Neurol. (Chicago) v.53, p.134, 1996;/ cited in Proc. Natl. Acad. Sci. USA, v.98, No.6, p.3440, 3/13/01

[119] East Boston Study, Arch. Neurol. (Chicago) v.54, p.1399, 1997/ cited in Proc. Natl. Acad. Sci. USA, v.98, No.6, p.3440, 3/13/01

[120] Neuropsychologia v.45, No.2, February 2007

[121] JAMA v.296 p.2805, 12/20/06

who received cognitive training had less of a decline in certain thinking skills than their peers who did not have training, and that some of the benefits of short-term cognitive training persisted for as long as five years.

In another study, it was shown that people with Alzheimer's disease have a history of partaking in fewer activities, especially intellectual activities, during midlife. This research indicated that patients with Alzheimer's disease were less active in midlife in terms of intellectual activities, physical activities, and passive (not physical) activities than people who did not have Alzheimer's disease. This study also revealed that people who were relatively inactive (for intellectual, physical, and passive activities) had approximately a 250% increased risk of developing Alzheimer's disease! In particular, the researchers showed that *intellectual activities* were *most* protective against Alzheimer's disease. These researchers also hypothesized that education and continued intellectual stimulation generate more connections in the brain, which makes the brain more resistant to the effects of the disease. Numerous other studies show that intellectually engaging activities are protective over time against cognitive decline and that the frequency and intensity of intellectual activity is related to cognitive function. Not only is intellectual stimulation associated with enhanced cognitive functioning, but lack of intellectual activity is a risk factor for the development of Alzheimer's disease.[122]

Exercise and Aging

According to researchers, age-related muscle loss can be reversed at any age using *strength-training exercise.* Using strength-training/weight-lifting exercise, elderly women reversed the muscle loss associated with aging and regained muscle and bone while loosing fat.[123] Strength training not only increases muscle mass and strength, but also increases bone density, restores good balance, enhances sleep, and helps people to stay vital and independent as they age. High-intensity resistance exercise training has been shown to be a feasible and effective means of counteracting muscle weakness and physical frailty in very elderly people.[124]

---

[122] Proc. Natl. Acad. Sci. USA, v.98, No.6, p.3440, 3/13/01

[123] www.strongwomen.com

[124] New England Journal of Medicine v.330, p.1769, 6/23/94

While most elderly individuals will die from atherosclerosis, cancer, or dementia, for an increasing number of the healthy *oldest* people, the loss of muscle strength will determine their chances of living an independent life until death, and therefore greatly affect their quality of life. Age-related disability is characterized by generalized weakness, impaired mobility and balance, and poor endurance. When an older person becomes physically frail, the result is falls, fractures, impairment in activities of daily living, and loss of independence. Falls contribute to 40% of admissions to nursing homes. Loss of muscle strength is an important factor in the process of frailty. A sedentary lifestyle and decreased physical activity and disuse are important determinants of the decline in muscle strength. It was shown that supervised *resistance exercise training* (for 45 minutes, three times per week for 10 weeks) doubled muscle strength and significantly increased gait velocity and stair-climbing power in a study of 100 frail nursing home residents (average age 87 years). This demonstrates that frailty in the elderly is not an irreversible effect of aging and disease, but can be reduced and perhaps even prevented. It was also observed that among non-disabled elderly people, function of the lower-extremity of their bodies was a predictor of whether or not they will suffer future disability. This study concluded that prevention of frailty can be achieved only by exercise.[125]

The brain is also enhanced through exercise. Not only does exercise increase the vasculature and blood supply in the brain, but there are chemicals and growth factors in the brain whose levels are raised from *exercise*.[126] These chemicals or neurotrophic factors that are released from nerve cells during exercise help nerve cells resist illness or injury, prompt them to grow and multiply, and strengthen connections between nerve cells. One of these chemicals, called Brain Derived Growth Factor, is believed to prevent the connections between nerve cells from breaking down and also help them grow back. Not only do these chemicals promote learning and memory, but may also help the brain resist Alzheimer's and Parkinson's diseases.[127]

There are several of these brain chemicals that are protective to neurons including Brain Derived Neurotrophic Factor and other neurotrophins and growth factors, which are believed to promote the survival and differentiation of neurons and promote plasticity of nerves and synapses.[128] In fact, studies

---

[125] Science v.278, No.5337, p.419, 10/17/97

[126] The Journal of Neuroscience v.20, No.8, p.2926, 4//15/00

[127] Science News v.169, No.8, p.122, 2/25/06; Stealing Time: The New Science of Aging, Warshofsky, TV Books 1999 p.222

[128] Science v.295, No.5560, p.1651, 1729, 3/1/02; Science v.270, No.5236, p.593, 10/27/95

have shown that *exercise* increases the levels of certain growth factors in the areas of the brain involved in motor function, cognition, reasoning, thinking, and learning. When groups of healthy people of the same age were compared by a battery of cognitive (reasoning, memory, mental process) tests, the groups that exercised performed better cognitively than the groups that did not exercise.[129] Furthermore, two recent studies demonstrated that even moderate exercise, such as walking, protected the aging brain from cognitive decline and reduced the risk of developing dementia.[130]

Exercise is not only beneficial to our general health and well-being, but it will allow us to remain independent and enhance our cognitive abilities as we age, which will greatly enhance our quality of life.

Stress and Aging

When we are under stress there is a release of *stress* hormones in our bodies. These hormones cause the mobilization of glucose from storage into the bloodstream, an increase in heart rate and blood pressure, and a suspension of various long-term, energy consuming functions, such as digestion, growth, reproduction, tissue repair, and maintenance of the immune system. The chronic production of the stress hormone cortisol that occurs when the body is exposed to continual stress has also been linked to heart disease and upper respiratory infections.[131]

Exposing our bodies to long-term stress is also believed to cause aging in our brains, and can damage neurons in the parts of the brain involved in learning and memory. Prolonged exposure to stress leads to loss of neurons, particularly in the hippocampus, which is a region of the brain central to learning and memory.[132] In fact, it has been documented that sustained stress can damage the hippocampus. Glucocorticoids, which are a class of steroid hormones secreted from the adrenal gland during stress, are believed to be involved in this neurotoxicity and can also impair the capacity of hippocampal neurons to survive a variety of neurological diseases, such as stroke and seizure.[133]

---

[129] Stealing Time: The New Science of Aging, Warshofsky, TV Books 1999 p.222-223; Nature, 373, 109, (1995)Cotman

[130] Science News v.166, No.13, p.197, 9/25/04

[131] Science News v.156, No.10, p.158, 9/4/99

[132] Curr Opin Neurobiology, v.5, No.2, p.205, Apr.1995

[133] Sapolsky, Stanford Univ. Biomedical & Biological Sciences; http://sbrc.stanford.edu/phd/faculty/phd_fac_list/sapolsky.html

It is important to reduce stress in our lives, or at the very least, learn to not let unimportant issues affect us.

Antioxidants, Vitamins, and Aging

Oxygen is required for life, but its consumption generates free radicals, which damage and age our bodies. Oxygen radicals can affect numerous cellular processes in our bodies linked to aging and the development of age-related diseases. It is therefore thought that factors that increase resistance to oxidative stress should have anti-aging benefits.[134] The benefits of eating fruits and vegetables to enhance successful aging are being examined. Fruits and vegetables, with their abundance of vitamins, minerals, phytochemicals, free-radical fighting *antioxidants*, and other beneficial compounds can fight off diseases and enhance health, which can help to give us longer, healthier lives. Antioxidants such as vitamins C, E, and betacarotene, boost immune function and reduce the risk of cancer and heart disease. Free radicals can also damage the neurons in our brains. Because our brains are in constant use, we generate and accumulate oxygen, or free radicals, which can cause damage to our brain tissues.[135] Antioxidants found in fruits, vegetables, plant foods, and supplements can help protect neurons in the brain from damage by free radicals.

Optimizing nutrition, including a diet rich in fruits and vegetables, may also provide the most practical means to delay age-related cataract formation. While light and oxygen are necessary for the function of the eye, when they are present in excess or in uncontrolled circumstances, they appear to be related to the development of cataracts. Researchers believe that compromises of the function of the lens and retina with aging are exacerbated by depleted or diminished antioxidant reserves and other related affects.[136] A diet rich in fruits and vegetables and their antioxidants may be helpful in decreasing the risk of age-related cataract formation.

A vitamin also important to the very young as well as mature adults is vitamin D, which is found in few foods except salmon and fatty fish, and is made when ultraviolet B from the Sun hits the skin. Because of the concern about skin cancer, many of us, especially children and seniors, may not be

---

[134] Nature v.408, No.6809, p.239, 11/9/00

[135] Stealing Time: The New Science of Aging, Warshofsky, TV Books 1999 p.207-9

[136] American Journal of Clinical Nutrition v 62, p.1439, Dec.1995

getting enough vitamin D. Inadequate amounts of vitamin D can cause rickets (soft bones, enlarged hearts) in babies and children, bone fractures in the elderly, and may possibly be involved in cancer and autoimmune diseases.[137] Data also suggests a correlation between vitamin D and a lower risk of multiple sclerosis.[138] Vitamin D helps regulate calcium for bones, nerves, and heart. Talk to your doctor about whether you should take vitamin D supplements.[139]

Calorie Restriction and Aging

Calorie Restriction is a method that has been used to extend life in various species of animals resulting in the animals actually remaining healthier, more disease free, and physiologically younger at more advanced ages. Every species, including one-celled animals, worms, rodents, fish, rats, and monkeys, have been shown to live significantly longer by life-extensions that would compare to humans living to 150 or 160 years of age. Calorie-restricted animals show positive physiological changes during their extended life, so that they are not extending a feeble existence. For example, calorie-restricted monkeys have healthier blood pressures, healthier levels of cholesterol, better levels of HDLs and LDLs, lower triglycerides, and a lower risk of heart disease, stroke, cancer, and diabetes.[140] Research suggests that blocking the growth of fat cells and having lower body fat could extend life.[141] Calorie restriction combats oxidative damage and is effective in retarding aging and preventing diseases associated with aging.[142] Restricting calories also lowers body temperature. Researchers have been curious if lower body temperature lengthens an animal's life span, perhaps by reducing free radical damage to cells over a lifetime.[143] Other research has shown a connection between calorie restriction and mitochondria, which are energy-converting organelles that with age decrease in number and generate greater amounts of harmful free radicals believed to damage DNA. In one study people on calorie-restricted diets showed an increase in the number of mitochondria in muscle cells although a decrease in DNA damage, and an

[137] FASEB Journal July 2005/Science News v. 170, No.20, 11/11/06

[138] JAMA v.296, p.2832, 2006. http://jama.ama-assn.org/cgi/content/abstract/296/23/2832;
Journal of the American Dietetic Association v.106, Issue 3, p.418, March 2006

[139] Science v. 302, No. 5652, p.1886, 12/12/03

[140] Science News v.158, No.22 p.341, 11/25/00 and Science News v.151, No.11, p.162, 3/15/97;
Stealing Time, Warshofsky, TV Books 1999 p.103-116; also see http://www.walford.com/research.htm

[141] Science v. 304, No. 5678, p.1731, 6/18/04

[142] Nature v.408, No.6809, p.245, 11/9/00

[143] Science v.314, p.825, 11/3/06; Science News v.170, No.22, p.350, 11/25/06

increase in activity of genes related to mitochondrial function.[144] There is much research on why calorie restriction increases lifespan and keeps the body physiologically younger.

Calorie-restriction involves feeding animals a diet that is rich in nutrients but lower in calories than a normal diet. While reduced in calories, the quality of the diet is increased so that essential nutrients such as vitamins, minerals, and amino acids are not diminished, and there is no malnourishment. The benefits of calorie restriction appear to begin at about 10 percent restriction and increase until the restriction approaches 50 percent. The reason individuals in semi-starved populations in various parts of the world don't live longer is not that they are calorie restricted, but that they are malnourished.

Researchers have examined the changes in gene-expression that occur with aging, and how calorie restriction can affect these changes.[145] In one study researchers analyzed the molecular changes associated with aging in mice. Genetic analysis revealed that during normal aging there is a distinct gene-expression pattern that shows an apparent stress response and lower expression of metabolic and biosynthetic genes. Researchers found that there are four major gene classes that display changes as we age. They then found that 84% of these age-related gene classes were either completely or partially suppressed by calorie restriction. Researchers also found that at the molecular level, calorie-restricted mice appear to be biologically younger. It appears that calorie restriction reduces age-associated degradation. This protection from age associated degradation by calorie restriction is due to: increasing DNA repair; altering gene expression; depressing metabolic rate; reducing oxidative stress; increasing protein metabolism; increasing energy metabolism; increasing biosynthesis of fatty acids and DNA precursors; and decreasing macromolecular damage. This study demonstrates the positive effects of calorie restriction on a molecular level, and reveals a link between gene expression and our eating behavior patterns. Further research is continuing to home in on the effects of particular genes associated with aging that are influenced by calorie restriction in an effort to understand why significantly restricting calories extends life in nearly every species tested in the lab.[146]

---

[144] Science News v.171, No.10, p.147, 3/10/07

[145] Science v. 285, No. 5432, p.1390, 8/27/99

[146] Science v. 304, No. 5678, p.1731, 6/18/04

Alzheimer's Disease and Aging

Alzheimer's disease has been estimated to affect 25 to 45 percent of people age 85 and older; although, the disease can begin in the 60's. The basic challenge for Alzheimer's clinicians and researchers is to keep the brain healthy and prevent disease pathology during the early stages. While Alzheimer's disease becomes more common with age, it is not a normal part of aging. Alzheimer's disease is physically characterized by abnormal deposits of certain proteins in the brain, specifically beta-amyloid protein plaques and tau protein tangles. It is still not known if these abnormal protein manifestations actually cause the disease or are just present with the disease.[147]

Researchers are investigating protective strategies and therapeutic interventions for preserving brain function and warding off or pushing back the onset of Alzheimer's disease. Certain protective strategies seem to have a beneficial effect if they are used years before any disease is present.[148] Protective strategies under investigation include: education and intellectual stimulation; exercise; estrogen therapy used early (currently under investigation); statins (cholesterol-lowering drugs); non-steroidal anti-inflammatory drugs; omega-3 fatty acids; and antioxidant vitamins, namely E, C, Niacin, and other antioxidants found in fruits, vegetables, and the spice turmeric.[149] Lifestyle also plays an important role in warding off Alzheimer's disease, including *not being overweight*. Results of recent epidemiological studies as well as animal model investigations suggest that intellectual stimulation, education, and varied physical exercise reduce Alzheimer's disease risk and push back symptoms. Not surprisingly, television watching is associated with increased incidence of Alzheimer's disease.[150]

As described in several studies cited in the section above, *Education and Aging*, intellectual stimulation and education have a significant impact on delaying Alzheimer's disease and dementia. Researchers hypothesized that education and continued intellectual stimulation generate more connections in the brain, which makes the brain more resistant to the effects of the disease. Numerous studies show that intellectually engaging activities are

---

[147] Science News v.160, No.18, p.286-287, 11/3/01

[148] Science News v.165, No.19, p.296, 5/8/04

[149] omega-3 fatty acids Science News v.166, No.10, p.148, 9/4/04; NSAIDS Science v.302, No.5648, p.1215, 11/14/03; niacin Science News v.166, No.9, p.142, 8/28/04; turmeric The Journal of Neuroscience, 11/1/01, v.21, No.21, p.8370; turmeric BBC NEWS, Wed., 11/21/01

[150] Science v. 309, No. 5736, p 864, 8/5/05

protective over time against cognitive decline and that the frequency and intensity of intellectual activity is related to cognitive function. Not only is intellectual stimulation associated with enhanced cognitive functioning, but lack of intellectual activity is a risk factor for the development of Alzheimer's disease. Using a mouse model, a study found that short but repeated learning sessions can slow the development of two brain lesions, plaques and tangles, which are characteristics of Alzheimer's disease. The finding suggests that the elderly, by keeping their minds active, can help delay the onset of this degenerative disease.[151]

There is a connection between chronically high insulin levels in the blood and Alzheimer's disease. Chronically high insulin levels in the blood appear to cause the accumulation of beta-amyloid protein in the brain and therefore may play a role in Alzheimer's disease. Consistent with this finding is that people with Type II diabetes, which is characterized by high levels of insulin circulating in the blood, have an increased risk of Alzheimer's disease. Several studies have shown that people with Type II diabetes have twice the risk of developing the disease as non-diabetics.[152] Whether the increase in Alzheimer's disease is due to high blood insulin or other factors related to diabetes has not been proven as yet, but avoiding diabetes (as well as insulin resistance) will certainly reduce the significant diabetes-related risk factor for Alzheimer's disease. Another study showed that women who are overweight at age 70 (and in their 70s) have a higher risk of developing Alzheimer's disease and dementia than slimmer women. This study revealed that 70-year-old women who had a BMI of 29.3 had an increased risk of developing Alzheimer's disease, and that for every 1.0 unit increase in BMI at age 70, Alzheimer's disease risk increased by 36%! In addition, women who developed dementia between ages 79 and 88 years were overweight to a slightly smaller degree and had a higher than average BMI at age 70 of 27.7. A woman who is 5-foot-4 and weighs about 170 pounds has a BMI of 29.[153] A BMI of 30 or higher is considered obese, a BMI between 25 and 30 is overweight, and a BMI of approximately 19-25 is average.[154] (See Appendix 2: Body Mass Index.)

There are also specific drugs and treatments currently being used to treat the symptoms of Alzheimer's disease. Researchers have developed drugs to treat

---

[151] Journal of Neuroscience v.27, p.751, 1/24/06

[152] Science v..301, No.5629, p.40, 7/4/03

[153] Arch Intern Med. v.163, p.1524, 2003; USA TODAY 7/14/2003

[154] www.cdc.gov/nccdphp/dnpa/bmi/bmi-adult.htm

Alzheimer's, such as memantine, which was shown to slow the progression of symptoms in patients with moderately severe disease.[155] In addition, researchers have investigated targeting certain enzymes involved in the processes that allow the development of amyloid plaques, which build up in brains of Alzheimer's patients.[156] Other studies have investigated immunizing against Alzheimer's disease using a beta-amyloid protein to block the development of, and even destroy, existing amyloid plaques.[157] Even an antibiotic has been studied for its potential use in dissolving the amyloid plaques.[158] In addition, results from another study suggested there could be some connection between high cholesterol levels and the brain degeneration in Alzheimer's patients, which has sparked research into the possible use of cholesterol-lowering drugs to slow progression of the disease.[159] Other research on preventatives and treatments include: resveratrol, a compound found in grapes and red wine;[160] a concentrated component called epigallocatechin-3-gallate (EGCG) from green tea;[161] sufficient daily recommended allowance amounts of folates from oranges, legumes, leafy green vegetables and folic acid supplements;[162] omega-3 fatty acids found in fish such as mackerel, sardines and salmon;[163] exercise of body and mind;[164] and niacin, particularly from food sources.[165]

There is much hope that this disease will be understood and effectively treated in the future. Until then it is crucial to keep your body healthy through nutrition, exercise, and maintaining a healthy weight, and your brain well stimulated through frequent and intense intellectual activity.

---

[155] Science v.289, No.5478, p.375, 7/21/00

[156] Science v.286 No.5440, p650, 10/22/99

[157] Science v.285, No.5425, p.175, 7/9/99; Science News v.156, No.2, p.20, 7/10/99; Science v.289, No.5478, p.375, 7/21/00

[158] Science v.290, No.5495, p.1273, 11/17/00

[159] Science v.294 No.5542. p508-509 10/19/01

[160] Journal of Biological Chemistry November 11, 2005

[161] Journal of Neuroscience Sept. 21, 2005

[162] The Journal of the Alzheimer's Association Inaugural issue 2005

[163] Online issue of the Journal of Neuroscience March 23, 2005

[164] Cell v.120, p.701, 3/11/05

[165] Neurol Neurosurg Psychiatry v.75, p.1093, 2004

Final Thoughts on Aging

Unless you are stricken with a disease in spite of your efforts to ward it off, there is absolutely no reason for your mind and body to significantly deteriorate. You may decline somewhat as you push through the century mark, but if you keep your mind and body young and healthy through good nutrition, exercise, and maintaining a healthy weight, as well as reducing stress, getting enough sleep, and continuing to stimulate your brain through intellectual pursuits, you can stay young mentally and physically well into old age. Find something that interests you, such as learning a foreign language, learning to play a musical instrument, learning to play chess, becoming an amateur astronomer, becoming a world traveler, or taking classes in subjects that you find fascinating. Curiosity may have killed the cat, but it will keep us young!

Knowing that our habits and behaviors can increase our chances of having a longer healthier life should further motivate us to take care of our minds and bodies now.

Epilogue

"Isabelle, that is the most beautiful wedding dress I have ever seen!" Sandy said, reaching over to touch a delicate pearl on Isabelle's light cream-colored dress.

"That slim-fitting maid-of-honor dress looks beautiful on your new figure, Sandy. I am so glad we could celebrate your reaching your weight-loss goal at the same time as my wedding, and have it all happen here in Tahiti – in this tropical paradise!" Isabelle said holding out her hands toward the window.

"Isabelle, don't stand too near the window, I can see that cute Trevor hunk of yours down on the beach in his tux – you know it's bad luck for the groom to see the bride right before the ceremony," Josie said flicking her hair over her shoulder as she looked down at the shimmering water. "This is a great spot – how did you find it?"

"Isabelle came down here to Tahiti to celebrate reaching her weight-loss goal, and she called me from this very phone!" Sandy said pointing at the phone on the bedside table of Isabelle's tropically-decorated hotel room. "Now, here we all are looking slim and svelte thanks to Isabelle and her 3:00 PM Secret! Look at those cute guys down there talking to Trevor." Sandy pointed down at the beach. "Are those Trevor's friends? If not, we should invite them to the wedding."

Josie ignored the men. "I stopped skipping breakfast and then raiding the pastry cart, and you, Jane, changed your New Year's resolution to include the ten-minute workout – and we all gave up being slaves to eating at night and staying up late in front of the boob tube wasting our lives away. I'm really glad we have all gotten to know each other so well this past year. I think we have each changed a lot – I know I have," Josie said thoughtfully, scanning her small group of friends, finally resting her eyes on Isabelle. Her mood lightened as she and Jane finally noticed the men Sandy was watching on the beach.

Ellen walked over to the window to see what everyone was looking at so intently. "I got rid of my idiot box, too. And without being a slave to the dinner routine, I have evenings free to go to the gym or library, and to take art history classes. Not only that, I have been getting eight hours of sleep at night and feel great!"

"You look great, Ellen. In fact, you all look great!" Madeline said smiling at her fellow bridesmaids. "After finally losing those 30 pounds I had been trying to shed for what felt like my whole life, Howard recently informed me he is rewarding me with a trip around the world starting with your wedding, Isabelle, here in Tahiti. After we return home from our travels we are enrolling in classes in oceanography together and plan to get a boat and live on it part of the time!" Madeline beamed with enthusiasm.

"Isn't Trevor's back-to-school focus on oceanography or marine biology or something similar?" Josie asked with her eyes still transfixed on the men.

"We're both going back to school – Trevor's in a PhD program in biology with an emphasis in zoology, and I've always been interested in geology, so I plan to start with basic science and math classes. At least with my accounting degree, I have some elementary math skills." Isabelle was nervously combing her hair for at least the tenth time.

"Yikes, math and science, that's pretty brave of you Isabelle. I knew you were thinking about going back to school, but you're not 18 any more." Jane turned her eyes from the men outside to look admiringly at Isabelle.

"Isabelle is still a youngster, Jane," Madeline said. "You are never too old to learn a new field or embark on a new adventure – otherwise you begin to die. I had wasted so much of my life waddling around uninspired, stuffing my dreams so far inside me I forgot I ever had any. Now, for the first time in my life I am slim, fit, and strong. I am rediscovering my dreams and honoring God with self-discipline and a body ready for anything He may lead me to do. Right now it's learning a little about the world and the oceans." Madeline's serious tone caught the attention of her younger friends.

"Madeline is right, we are all fit and strong, and have freed ourselves of our self-destructive, immobilizing lifestyles." Sandy held up her teacup. "Let's all toast Isabelle and Trevor's new and exciting life together. And let's also toast all of our new bodies and our upcoming adventures as we all pursue and realize our dreams, our destinies!"

"Hear hear!" the women all chimed in with enthusiasm.

At last I am free
A body fit for my dreams
And my destiny…

Isabelle

It may be worth mentioning that eating is not primarily about answering hunger pangs and pleasing the palate, though it is usually talked about in those terms. The primary purpose is to nourish and fuel the body and all its organs. Finding and selecting foods that will do this effectively and without causing harmful side effects requires accurate knowledge of their contents and nutritional benefits.

To assist you in making optimal food choices, I have included this Appendix, which explains and supports the nutritional guidelines given in *The Ten Tips for Good Nutrition* and *What Foods to Emphasize on 3:00 PM Days and Free Days* in Chapter 3. The sections include what you need to know about vegetables, fruits, plant foods, fats, proteins, sugars and carbohydrates, as well as vital information on food allergies and intolerance. It also highlights many surprising findings of nutrition research.

Before proceeding with the Appendix, I would like to mention the benefits of choosing **organic foods over non-organic foods**, and cite a few reasons why it is worth the extra dollars to buy organic. Organic versions of dairy, meat, and produce are available in many supermarkets and health food stores and will help you avoid consuming hormones and pesticides. Researchers have learned that women with elevated levels of pesticides in their breast tissue have a greater breast cancer risk. Perhaps this is because the molecular structure of some pesticides closely resembles that of estrogen and these molecules may attach to the estrogen receptor sites in the body.[166] There is also an insulin-like growth factor (IGF-1) that promotes breast cancer, as well as prostate and colon cancers. In the United States, cows are injected with the bovine growth hormone, rBGH, which causes a natural growth factor, IGF-1, to be released into the body of the cow. Cows injected with rBGH have been found to have unusually high levels of IGF-1 in their fat and milk. IGF-1 has growth-promoting effects, it does not break down during pasteurization and digestion, and is absorbed from the gastrointestinal tract into the body. Studies have suggested that excess IGF-1 levels in rBGH milk is a risk factor for breast and colon cancers.[167] Another study showed a positive correlation between circulating IGF-I concentration in the blood and risk of breast cancer among premenopausal women.[168] The role of IGF-1 in cancer is supported by epidemiologic studies, which have found that high levels of circulating IGF-I are associated with increased risk of several common cancers, including those of the prostate, breast, colorectum, and lung.[169] I believe spending a few extra dollars on organic foods in order to preserve my health is well worth it.

The information in Chapter 3 and this Appendix explain why it is so important to eat healthy foods, and is intended as a reference and guide as you sort out the food choices that work best for you.

---

[166] http://www.mayoclinic.com/health/breast-cancer-prevention/WO00091

[167] Journal of the National Cancer Institute v.93, No.3, p.238, 2/7/01

[168] The Lancet v.351, Issue 9113, p.1393, 5/9/98

[169] Journal of the National Cancer Institute v.92, No.18, p.1472, 9/20/00

Vegetables, Fruits, and Plant-Based Foods

The U.S. Departments of Agriculture and Health and Human Services suggest eating 3 to 5 servings of vegetables and 2 to 4 servings of fruits every day.[170] Hundreds of research studies have demonstrated the beneficial health effects of eating fruits and vegetables, and that a diet rich in fruits, vegetables, and plant-based foods lowers the risk of developing cancer and other diseases.

There are many different highly beneficial *vegetables* that should be eaten daily. Try to select a variety of fresh vegetables, especially deeply colored ones, including broccoli, spinach, cauliflower, chard, kale, mustard greens, turnips, rutabaga, carrots, beets, radishes, green and purple cabbage, parsley, various sprouts and sea vegetables, onions, garlic, asparagus, Brussels sprouts, and red and green peppers.

Fruit should also be part of your daily diet and can be eaten whole or in fruit salads. Whole fruits include grapefruit, oranges, tangerines, apples, lemons, figs, papaya, pineapple, mangos, blueberries, strawberries, raspberries, tomatoes, bananas, apricots, peaches, plums, apples, cantaloupe, cherries, pears, grapes, and kiwis. Fruits can also be consumed in nutritional shakes and smoothies that can be made from some combination of foods such as soy, vegetable and/or nut powders, yogurt, fresh or frozen bananas, blueberries, strawberries, raspberries, peaches, apricots, apples, and wheat germ.

Because many people don't eat adequate servings of vegetables and fruits, regularly drinking vegetable and lower-sugar fruit *juices* can provide many of the nutrients you need to maximize health. Even though juicing does not give you all of the fiber, it is much better to assure yourself you are getting the nutrients you need when you find you are not eating sufficient vegetables and fruits every day. If you don't have time to juice, there are often juice bars or juice stands in health-food stores and health-food restaurants. Fresh juices can be made with spinach, carrots, apples, grapefruit, and combinations of a variety of fruits and vegetables. Drinking fresh vegetable juice regularly is a good insurance policy for a more healthy and energetic life.

---

[170] www.metlife.com

If you are not a big fan of vegetables, then combine them with foods you enjoy eating. For example, spinach is easy to eat and can be added to almost any meal or eaten alone. Fresh spinach is not only packed with nutrients, but it also tastes good. You can add spinach leaves to almost everything you eat. For example, if you hate salad but love enchiladas, then cut an enchilada into sections and put it on a large bed of spinach (and eat the spinach). The natural chemicals that are contained in fruits and vegetables are known fighters of cancer and other diseases. To illustrate the importance of including a variety of fruits and vegetables in your daily diet, I will list some plant foods, vital compounds, their benefits, and associated colors.

Vegetables and fruits are believed to slow or prevent the onset of chronic diseases because they are rich sources of a variety of nutrients including vitamins, trace minerals, dietary fiber, and many other classes of biologically active compounds including *phytochemicals*. Phytochemicals may act in concert with each other by regulating detoxification enzymes, stimulating the immune system, reducing platelet aggregation, regulating cholesterol synthesis and hormone metabolism, reducing blood pressure, and being involved with antioxidant, antibacterial, and antiviral effects.[171]

Different phytochemicals are associated with the colors of various fruits, vegetables, and legumes. The color green contains the phytochemicals thiocyanates, indoles, lutein, zeaxanthin, sulforaphane, and isothicyanates; yellow contains limonene; orange contains carotenes; red contains lycopene; purple, orange and red contain resveratrol, ellagic acid, cyaniding, and quercetin; brown contains genistein, phytosterols, and saponins; and white contains allium, allyl sulfide, and quercetin.[172] All of these phytochemicals are important, so it is beneficial to eat a variety of colors of fruits, vegetables, and *legumes* in order to get an array of beneficial compounds.

Every different vegetable has its own unique combination of important and highly beneficial nutrients. For example, consider the variety of nutrients in the following: *Spinach* is a good source of antioxidants and phytochemicals including lutein, beta-carotene and zeaxanthin, B-vitamins including folacin (or folic acid), magnesium, and potassium. *Broccoli* is a good source of antioxidants and phytochemicals including indoles and sulforaphane, beta-carotene, lutein, vitamin C, phytosterols, folic acid, and minerals such as zinc, chromium, selenium, calcium, magnesium, phosphorous and potassium.

---

[171] American Journal of Clinical Nutrition v.70, No.3, p.475, September 1999

[172] The Omega Diet, Artemis P. Simopoulos, M.D., and Jo Robinson, HarperPerennial 1999, p.135

Carrots are a good source of antioxidants and phytochemicals, including vitamin C, beta-carotene and other carotinoids, selenium, folacin and other B vitamins, minerals including calcium and potassium, and calcium pectate (a soluble fiber). *Dulse*, a sea vegetable, is a good source of vitamin B12, trace minerals, calcium, potassium, chromium, antioxidants and phytochemicals including alginate, vitamins C, E and K, and beta-carotene. *Sprouts* including alfalfa, radish and sunflower sprouts, as well as sprouted beans and grains such as wheat berries, lentils, chickpeas (garbanzos), green peas, flax, and pinto beans, are a good source of antioxidants and phytochemicals, beta-carotene, vitamin C, trace minerals, and protein. Reading through the above listed array of beneficial nutrients in different fruits and vegetables with their diverse colors illustrates the importance of variety. Eating a combination of these different foods provides a range of health-promoting nutrients.

Fruits have numerous health benefits. *Figs*, for example, are a good source of calcium, potassium, zinc, trace minerals, antioxidants, phytochemicals, enzymes, vitamin A, pectin fiber, and a digestive enzyme called ficin. *Grapefruit* is a good source of vitamin C, bioflavinoids, antioxidants and phytochemicals, including beta-carotene, lycopene, quercetic and courmarins, galacteronic acid, citrus pectin, and minerals. Just as with vegetables, it is important to eat a variety of fruits.

Different fruits and vegetables have specific combinations of benefits in our bodies. *Blueberries* and other deeply colored fruits and vegetables contain pigments called *flavonoids* that are high in *antioxidant activity*. In fact, blueberries as well as strawberries and spinach were found to enhance memory and motor coordination in aging rats.[173] Mental ability of the rats was compared after they were fed food supplemented with blueberries, strawberries, spinach, and food with no supplement (the control group). All rats receiving supplemented food performed better on memory tests, and the blueberry-supplemented group also demonstrated notable improvement over the control group in tests of motor coordination. In fact, older blueberry-supplemented rats outperformed unsupplemented younger rats, which suggests reversals in age related declines. Chemical-signaling characteristics in the rat's brains were also measured in an area of the brain involved in coordination, and each supplement (blueberries, strawberries and spinach) showed a different benefit pattern in the brain. The rat's ages in the studies would compare to humans in their sixties, and the amount of blueberries consumed would compare to a cup a day for humans.

---

[173] Science News v. 156 No. 12 p. 180, 9/18/99

The benefits of vegetables, fruits, and soy have been carefully analyzed.[174] Researchers found that plant foods are full of phytochemicals, which contribute to good health and the suppression of disease. Risk of cardiovascular disease, macular degeneration, and prostate, esophageal and other cancers can be reduced or prevented by carotenoids such as lycopene found in tomatoes and leutein found in spinach and kale. Various cancers have been shown to be prevented or ameliorated by glucosinolates such as glucoraphanin found in broccoli. Phenolics such as resveratrol found in red grapes and red wine have been shown to improve or prevent cardiovascular disease and cancers. Phytoestrogens such as genistein and daidzein found in soybeans, tofu and soy products have been shown to ameliorate or prevent cardiovascular disease, osteoporosis, and breast, prostate and colon cancers. In addition, the compounds in garlic are well known to have beneficial qualities including protective effects against stomach and colorectal cancers,[175] as well as beneficial effects in cardiovascular disease.[176]

Nutrients found in fruits and vegetables also contain many important vitamins and minerals, such as vitamin C and the B vitamin folic acid. A study suggested that *vitamin C* taken in amounts approximating several grams per day, may lessen the body's response to stress with respect to the chronic production of the hormone cortisol.[177] Chronic cortisol production has been linked to heart disease and upper respiratory infections. Also, eating vitamin C rich foods appears to increase the production of the IgG antibody in rats, which is a measure of immune-system function. Vitamin C rich foods include red and green peppers, broccoli, oranges, apples, grapefruit, Brussels sprouts, strawberries, and papaya.

Folic acid has been found to benefit the heart and reduce the risk of heart attacks. Research suggests that intake of folate and vitamin B_6 above the current recommended dietary allowance may be important in the primary prevention of coronary heart disease among women.[178] In the Harvard Nurses Heath Study, it was found that women who consumed an average of 400 micrograms of folic acid and 3 milligrams of vitamin B6 per day were about 50 percent less likely to suffer a heart attack than those who consumed only a small amount of these vitamins. Folic acid supplementation improved

---

[174] Science v. 285, No. 5426, p. 377, 7/16/99

[175] American Journal of Clinical Nutrition v. 72, No. 4, p.1047, October 2000

[176] American Journal of Clinical Nutrition v.34, p.2100, 1981

[177] Science News v. 156 No.10 p.158, 9/4/99

[178] JAMA v.279, p359, 1998

cognitive performance in older adults.[179] Research has demonstrated that folic acid deficiency causes breaks in chromosomes, which contain DNA, and that folic acid supplements can prevent such breaks.[180] Folic acid supplements are recommended for pregnant women, according to the U. S. Food and Drug Administration.[181] The U.S. Public Health Service recommended in September 1992 that all women of childbearing age should consume 400 micrograms of folic acid daily to reduce the risk of having their child affected with spina bifida and other neural tube defects. In 1998 the FDA also mandated that U.S. manufacturers must fortify grain-based foods with folic acid. In addition, the CDC recommended that women who can get pregnant should consume 400 micrograms of folic acid every day.[182] The FDA also stated that adequate levels of folic acid, in the form of folate, can be obtained from natural food sources. Rich sources of folic acid include vegetables, especially spinach and other dark-green leafy vegetables, citrus and other fruits, beans and legumes, whole grains, and certain breakfast cereals. Women can also assure adequate intake by taking dietary supplements containing folic acid. Total daily folic acid intake, however, should be less than 1 milligram.

Legumes, *dry beans*, and *soybeans* are high in nutrients and low in fat, and are excellent sources of protein, dietary fiber, and a variety of micronutrients and phytochemicals. Studies show that dry bean intake has the potential to decrease serum cholesterol concentrations, improve many aspects of the diabetic state, and provide metabolic benefits that aid in weight control. Soybeans are a unique source of the isoflavones, genistein, and diadzein, which have numerous biological functions. Soy foods and isoflavones have received attention for their potential role in preventing and treating cancer, including breast and prostate, as well as osteoporosis. Studies have demonstrated that many natural constituents of plants, in particular soy, can lower cholesterol concentrations and may improve other aspects of vascular health.[183] Isoflavone proteins, sometimes referred to as phytoestrogens or plant estrogens, in soy are also currently being investigated for their ability to protect cholesterol from oxidation. The "bad" cholesterol, or low-density lipoproteins (LDL's), become dangerous when they are oxidized, after which they can transform into the constituents of plaque, which can clog arteries.

---

[179] The Lancet v.369 No.9557, p.208, January 2007

[180] Science News v.156, No.19, p.293, 11/6/99

[181] Office of Public Affairs Fact Sheet 2/29/96, http://vm.cfsan.fda.gov/~dms/wh-folic.html

[182] Science News v.165, No.22, p.349, 5/29/04

[183] Science News v.153, No.22, p.349, 5/30/98

Soybeans and soy foods may have many health-promoting effects, including cholesterol reduction, improved vascular health, preserved bone mineral density, and reduced menopausal symptoms. Soy may also have beneficial effects on renal function and some cancers.[184] For example, men who eat soy-rich diets have a lower risk of prostate cancer.[185] Studies supporting soy consumption for breast cancer include data suggesting that both isoflavones and other soy constituents may exert cancer-preventive effects in post-menopausal women by altering estrogen metabolism away from genotoxic metabolites toward inactive metabolites,[186] and results suggesting that high intake of certain phytoestrogens may reduce the risk of breast cancer.[187] Another study concluded that a soy-containing diet in adult women provides little or no protection from breast cancer, but may be beneficial if consumed in early life before puberty or during adolescence. Also, no negative effects of soy on breast cancer have been observed.[188] Other research found that some phytoestrogenic compounds, at the levels consumed in the typical American-style diet, are associated with reduced risk of endometrial cancer.[189] Finally, the antioxidant action of soy compounds may be significant with regard to risk of atherosclerosis, cardiovascular disease in general, and cancer.[190] Overall, the consumption of soy generally has been considered beneficial, nevertheless because of their estrogenic activity, negative effects of isoflavones have been postulated and there has been some controversy. Some researchers reviewing the literature concluded that isoflavones as typically consumed in diets based on soy or containing soy products are safe.[191]

There are hundreds of studies demonstrating the benefits of various plant foods that can be easily found in science, medical, and nutrition journals. So please try to incorporate these foods into your daily diet. It is difficult not to notice that there is controversy and ongoing studies in research on nutrition and science in general. We have to do the our best to read all information and give weight to research that is performed by reputable, unbiased researchers in a rigorous manner. In addition to that, we should use common sense.

---

[184] American J. of Clinical Nutrition v.70, No.3, p.464, Sept 1999; American J. of Clinical Nutrition v.70, No.3, p.439, Sept 1999

[185] Science News v.156, No.19, p.295, 11/6/99

[186] Cancer Epidemiol Biomarkers Prev. v.9, No.8, p. 781, Aug 2000

[187] Cancer Epidemiol Biomarkers prev v.11, No.9, p.815, Sept 2002

[188] J Steroid Biochem Mol Biol v.83(1-5), p.113, Dec 2002

[189] J Natl Cancer Inst v.95, No.15, p.1158, Aug 6, 2003

[190] American Journal of Clinical Nutrition v.72, No.2, p.395, Aug 2000

[191] Nutrition Reviews v.61, No.1, p.1-33, Jan 2003

Fats

Fats are the primary components of our brains, nervous system, cell membranes, eyes, adrenal glands, and male testes. Fats are involved in vital functions in our bodies including the synthesis of hormones and maintenance of nerves, skin, cell membranes, nervous system, brain, and mucous membranes. They are also involved in healthy functioning of the immune, reproductive, cardiovascular, endocrine, digestive, and central nervous systems. Fats facilitate oxygen transportation, stabilize blood sugar, and are involved in absorption of calcium and the fat-soluble vitamins (A, D, E, and K). They also influence blood pressure and affect inflammation, allergies, and pain sensitivity. Fats are an important part of a healthy diet, and avoiding all types of fats is not the way to slim down.

The low-fat, low-protein, high-carbohydrate diets that have been popular for years have robbed many people of the essential amino acids found in proteins and the *essential fatty acids* found in *fats*. These diets also result in the discharge of too much sugar into the bloodstream. In an attempt to cut non-beneficial fats from our diets, people have ended up cutting the healthy essential fats and proteins as well. Many of these low-fat diets have also inadvertently encouraged the consumption of harmful *transfats* (discussed later in this section). Research is pointing toward the importance of making healthy fats and oils part of our diet. Whether you consume generous amounts of fats and oils in your diet, or eat relatively little fat, it is important to eat essential and beneficial fats, such as olive oil, fish and fish oils, flaxseed oil, nuts, seeds, avocados, and canola oil.

During the past fifty years the percentage of overweight Americans has increased dramatically while the consumption of fat as a percentage of our diet has decreased. This is not what many people would expect. Interestingly, during this same time sugar consumption has increased dramatically. Ironically, in a study done a number of years ago it was shown that fatty acid synthesis within the body was actually stimulated by a low-fat, high-carbohydrate diet, whereas there was minimal fatty acid synthesis in people eating a high-fat diet.[192] Other studies have also shown the stimulation of fatty acid synthesis by low-fat, high-carbohydrate diets.[193]

---

[192] J Clin Invest v.97, p.2081, 1996

[193] Proceedings of Society for Experimental Biology and Medicine v.225, p.178, 2000; J of Lipid Research v.41, p.595, Apr 2000

An analysis of the low-fat diet phenomenon[194] revealed that while hundreds of millions of dollars have been spent to support the theory that low-fat diets are beneficial, the research has failed to prove that eating a low-fat diet will help us live longer. Since the early 1970s, the average intake of fat in America has decreased from over 40% of total calories to 34%, yet the incidence of heart disease has not decreased. While death from heart disease has decreased, it is believed to be primarily because doctors are treating heart disease more successfully as medical procedures have improved. Obesity and diabetes (which both increase heart disease risk) have increased since the low-fat phenomenon began. While there are positive effects from lowering fat, these effects seem to be counteracted by a high intake of carbohydrates. It was also concluded from a fifteen-year study by the World Cancer Research Fund and the American Institute for Cancer Research that there is neither "convincing" or "probable" reasons to believe that dietary fat causes cancer. In addition, low-fat diets are generally by definition excessively high-carbohydrate diets, which can raise triglyceride and LDL (bad) cholesterol, lower HDL (good) cholesterol, and cause insulin resistance and *Syndrome X*, which is associated with heart disease.[195] (See discussion in the Sugars and Carbohydrates section later in this Appendix on page 141.)

There is a growing trend away from the extreme high-carbohydrate diets toward a more balanced diet. Many doctors and nutritionists are recommending reducing sugars and carbohydrates and emphasizing a more balanced approach to eating.

Where to Find Good Fats

Essential fatty acids are a key part of a healthy diet. The *essential fatty acids* include the *omega-3* and *omega-6* fats and are required by the body. In order to maintain a healthy body, we must consume essential fatty acids as well as the essential amino acids found in proteins.

> The essential *omega-3* fatty acids are found in flaxseed oil; fish oil; cold-water and fatty fish including salmon, tuna, cod, halibut, anchovy and shrimp; flaxseeds; pumpkin seeds; walnuts; canola oil; dark green leafy vegetables; sea vegetables; soybeans; wheat germ; and sprouts. Flaxseed oil and fish are the richest sources.

---

[194] Science v.291, No.5513, p.2536, 3/30/01

[195] Science v.291, No.5513, p.2536, 3/30/01; Syndrome X first described by Dr. Gerald Reaven of Stanford University

The essential *omega-6* fatty acids are found in evening primrose oil, raw nuts and seeds, legumes, leafy green vegetables, meats, grains, borage oil, black currant seed oil, gooseberry oils, and grapeseed oil. Vegetable oils, such as corn, safflower, sunflower, soybean, cottonseed, and sesame also contain omega-6 fatty acids, although these oils are generally processed and hydrogenated and should be avoided as they contain transfats (discussed below in the omega-6 subsection).

The *monounsaturated fatty acids*, also called *omega-9* fatty acids, are not essential but have tremendous health benefits. Good sources of monounsaturated fats include olive oil, canola oil, avocados, and nuts such as almonds, pistachios, pecans, cashews, hazelnuts, macadamia nuts, and peanuts.

Most people consume a lot more omega-6 than omega-3 so it is important to emphasize omega-3 rich foods such as fish and flaxseed oil or take supplements.

What Are Fats and Why Are They Necessary?

Fats are composed of one to three fatty acids, a glycerol molecule, and an alcohol molecule, and are made up of carbon, oxygen, and hydrogen atoms. Fats are categorized in part by the number of fatty acids they possess, such as *mono-, di-, and tri-*glycerides. Fats are further categorized as *saturated fats* and as *unsaturated fats*, which are in the forms of *mono-unsaturated* and *poly-unsaturated*. *Saturated fats* have all possible hydrogen atoms present with their carbon atoms, which means that the chains of carbon atoms in these molecules have single bonds between them, and hydrogen atoms also bonded to each carbon atom. Saturated fats are generally solid at room temperature and are found in fats of beef, pork, lamb, organ meats, and dairy products, as well as in coconut oil, palm oil, and cocoa butter. *Unsaturated fats* possess a number of double bonds along their carbon-atom chains between some of the carbon atoms, and therefore do not have all possible hydrogen atoms present. Unsaturated fats are liquid at room temperature. *Mono-unsaturated fats* include the beneficial *omega-9* oils and *poly-unsaturated fats* include the *essential omega-3* and *omega-6* oils. Omega-3 fatty acids have their first double bond after the third carbon atom and omega-6 fatty acids have their first double bond after the sixth carbon atom.

Cholesterol is a soft, waxy substance that the body manufactures. It is a component of cell membranes and is essential for production of many hormones, vitamin D, and bile acids. Cholesterol is found in all parts of the body including the brain and nervous system as well as skin, muscle, heart, liver, intestines, and skeleton. Our blood cholesterol levels are affected by the amount of cholesterol our bodies produce as well as the cholesterol and saturated fats in the foods we eat. Cholesterol is carried in lipoproteins, which are formed in the liver. *Low-density lipoproteins (LDLs)* carry most of the cholesterol from the liver into the body and, if not removed from the blood, can cause cholesterol and fat build up in the arteries contributing to atherosclerosis. Cholesterol is also carried in *high-density lipoproteins (HDLs)* back to the liver for processing or removal from the body. HDLs are often called "good" cholesterol because they help remove unneeded cholesterol from the blood thereby reducing cholesterol and fat build up in the arteries.

Within the body, fat cells perform different functions. Some fat cells surround vital organs, cushion the spinal cord, and burn calories for heat by the process of thermogenesis, which maintains body heat. Other fat cells furnish an insulating layer beneath the skin, which provides warmth for the body and stored fat for future energy requirements. Fats are important in the diet because they supply the essential fatty acids, provide energy, and are involved in the synthesis of hormones and the maintenance of nerves, skin, cell membranes, nervous system, brain, and mucous membranes. They also facilitate oxygen transportation, absorption of calcium and fat-soluble vitamins A, D, E, and K, and help to stabilize blood sugar. When fats are eaten, they cause the release of the hormone *cholecystokinin (CCK)*, which sends a message to the brain that your body has reached *satiety*, which makes you feel full and therefore signals you to stop eating.

Fatty acids that we eat are also converted to other necessary fatty acids and compounds within our bodies. Two primary fatty acids of the omega-3 and omega-6 groups are *alpha-linolenic acid (LNA)*, which is an *omega-3* fatty acid, and *linoleic acid (LA)*, which is an *omega-6* fatty acid. These two fatty acids are transformed in our bodies into other compounds that are essential for healthy functioning of our bodies. For example:

1. The *omega-3 family of fatty acids* are transformed in the body such that the *omega-3 fatty acid alpha-linolenic acid (LNA)* is converted

into *eicosapentaenoic acid (EPA)*, which is then converted into *docosahexaenoic acid (DHA)*. EPA and DHA are further converted into the omega-3 family of *eicosanoid* hormones.

2. The *omega-6 family of fatty acids* are transformed in the body such that the *omega-6 fatty acid linoleic acid (LA)* is converted into *gamma-linolenic acid (GLA)*, which is then converted into *arachidonic acid (AA)*. AA and GLA are further converted into the omega-6 family of *eicosanoid* hormones.[196]

The transformed fatty acids, EPA, DHA, GLA, and AA, can also be obtained directly from certain foods.

Essential fatty acids including *EPA, DHA, GLA*, and *AA* are necessary for the production of *prostaglandins* and other *eicosanoid* hormones. These hormones are required for healthy functioning of certain systems in our bodies including the immune, reproductive, cardiovascular, endocrine, digestive, and central nervous systems. They also influence blood pressure and affect inflammation, allergies, and pain sensitivity. The functions of the hormones from the omega-3 and omega-6 families are believed to have certain opposite effects. For example, omega-6 eicosanoids are suspected to be more pro-inflammatory whereas the omega-3 eicosanoids have a counteracting anti-inflammatory effect.[197] See following two subsections on omega-3 fatty acids and omega-6 fatty acids.

Benefits of Omega-3 Fatty Acids

Beneficial effects of the omega-3 fatty acids have been demonstrated in coronary heart disease, hypertension, Type II diabetes, renal disease, rheumatoid arthritis, ulcerative colitis, Crohn's disease, and chronic obstructive pulmonary disease, and may generally be helpful in lowering the risk or lessening the severity of inflammatory and autoimmune diseases.[198] Researchers are delving into the biochemical reasons for the health-promoting effects of omega-3 fatty acids. For example, the anti-inflammatory benefits of omega-3 fatty acids are at least in part due to its effect on the

---

[196] The Omega Diet, Artemis P. Simopoulos, M.D., and Jo Robinson, HarperPerennial 1999, p.40

[197] The Omega Diet, Artemis P. Simopoulos, M.D., and Jo Robinson, HarperPerennial 1999, p.43

[198] American Journal of Clinical Nutrition v.70, No.3, 560, September 1999

membrane lipid composition of our cells and their reaction to inflammatory stimuli.[199]

The omega-3 fatty acids are believed to reduce the incidence of clogged arteries, lower the rate of synthesis of triglycerides by the liver, and lower blood pressure. Flaxseed oil, a rich source of omega-3 fatty acids, has been studied for its beneficial effects on lowering blood cholesterol and LDL (bad cholesterol) levels while raising HDL (good cholesterol) levels, normalizing high blood pressure, and improving circulatory problems. In addition, research suggests there may be protection against the risk of digestive tract cancers with fish consumption.[200]

Dietary intake of the omega-3 fatty acid alpha-linolenic acid (LNA), a precursor to EPA and DHA, has been investigated for its potential in lowering the risk of fatal *heart disease*. Experimental studies on laboratory animals and humans suggest that LNA may reduce the risk of arrhythmia. One study demonstrated the protective effects of higher intake of dietary LNA against fatal heart disease in women.[201] It has also been reported that an omega-3 fatty acid-rich Mediterranean diet seems to be more efficient than currently-used diets in the prevention of coronary events and death.[202] Eskimos, who eat an abundance of the omega-3 fatty acids *EPA* and *DHA* in the form of cold-water *fish,* were found to have an unusually low incidence of coronary heart disease. In fact, numerous studies have demonstrated that fish consumption is related to a reduced risk of coronary heart disease. Fish and fish oils have been shown to lower triglyceride levels and low-density lipoprotein cholesterol (bad cholesterol), inhibit platelet aggregation, and potentially reduce blood pressure.[203]

Epidemiologic data have been evaluated for the potential benefits of eating fish to reduce the risk of coronary heart disease. In one study, data from the Chicago Western Electric Study was used to examine the relation between fish consumption and a 30-year risk of death from coronary heart disease in 1822 men who were 40 to 55 years old and who had been free of cardiovascular disease. The data showed that fish consumption is related to a reduced risk of death from coronary heart disease.[204] Other research has

---

[199] Proc. Natl. Acad. Sci. USA, v.103, 15184, 2006/ Science v.314, p.567, 10/27/06

[200] American Journal of Clinical Nutrition v.70, No.1, 85, July 1999

[201] American Journal of Clinical Nutrition v.69, No.5, 890, May 1999

[202] Lancet v.343, No.8911, p1454, 6/11/94

[203] Science v.278, No.5345, p.1904, 12/12/97

[204] New England Journal of Medicine v.336, No.15, p.1046, 4/10/97

shown that a modest intake of fatty fish (two or three portions per week) may reduce mortality in men who have recovered from myocardial infarction.[205] Researchers have also examined the beneficial effects of omega-3 fatty acids on *blood pressure* and found that supplementation with omega-3 fatty acids found in fish oils may reduce blood pressure. One study showed that diet supplementation with a relatively high dose of omega-3 fatty acids can lead to clinically relevant blood pressure reductions in individuals with untreated hypertension.[206]

More recent finding and studies on the benefits of omega-fatty acids on cardiovascular health include: 1) Using a daily dose of 4 grams of a purified extract of omega-3 fatty acids from fish in patients with very high triglycerides reduced their triglycerides by an average of 45% and their very-low-density-lipoprotein cholesterol ("bad cholesterol") by more than 50%.[207] 2) Since there are currently about 400,000 deaths annually in the U.S. alone and millions more worldwide from fatal arrhythmias, and since there is considerable evidence from laboratory and clinical trials that omega-3 fatty acids of fish oil will prevent fatal arrhythmias, the antiarrhythmic actions of omega-3 fatty acids could have considerable potential public-health benefits.[208] 3) A recent literature review for the development of a dose-response relationship between fish consumption and stroke risk revealed that any fish consumption confers a substantial risk reduction in stroke compared to no fish consumption, with the possibility that additional consumption confers incremental benefits.[209] 4) European and American Cardiac Societies incorporated omega-3 fatty acids EPA and DHA into recent treatment guidelines for myocardial infarction, prevention of cardiovascular disease, treatment of ventricular arrhythmias and prevention of sudden cardiac death, and advise physicians to reduce the burden of cardiovascular disease by advocating EPA and DHA to all patients likely to benefit.[210]

Recent research into the benefits of omega-3 fatty acids on neurological, psychiatric, and cognitive conditions include the following: 1) The demonstrated benefits of omega-3 essential fatty acid supplementation in a variety of psychiatric disorders prompted a study finding that omega-3 fatty acid supplementation resulted in significantly greater improvements in

---

[205] Lancet v.2, No.8666, p.757, 9/30/89

[206] Arch Intern Med v.153, No.12, p.1429, 6/28/93

[207] Am J Health Syst Pharm v.64, No.6, p.595, Mar 2007

[208] Curr Opin Lipidol v.18, No.1, p.31, Feb 2007

[209] Am J Prev Med v.29, No.4, p.347, Nov 2005

[210] Curr Opin Clin Nutr Metab Care v.10, No.2, p.129, Mar 2007

depression, suicide, dealing with daily stresses, and well being, as well as achieving substantial reductions in indicators of suicidal behavior.[211]   2) Increasing evidence that fatty acid deficiencies or imbalances may contribute to childhood neurodevelopmental disorders prompted a recent study presenting preliminary evidence that omega-3 fatty acids may be an effective treatment for children with autism.[212]   3) Researchers found that fish intake was associated with a slower rate of the cognitive decline that normally occurs with age.[213]   4) A number of critical trials have confirmed the benefits of dietary supplementation with omega-3 fatty acids not only in several psychiatric conditions but also in inflammatory, autoimmune, and neurodegenerative diseases.[214]

The question of whether the risk due to potential contaminants in fish is overridden by the benefits of fish has been addressed by several studies including the following: 1) It was concluded that for major health outcomes among adults, based on both the strength of the evidence and the potential magnitudes of effect, the benefits of fish intake exceed the potential risks, even for women of childbearing age.[215]   2) One study found that maternal seafood consumption of less than 340 grams per week in pregnancy did not protect children from adverse outcomes, however, beneficial effects were evident on child development with maternal seafood intakes of more than 340 grams per week, suggesting that advice to limit seafood consumption could actually be detrimental and demonstrating that the risks from the loss of nutrients were greater than the risks of harm from exposure to trace contaminants in the 340 grams seafood eaten weekly.[216]   3) According to two recent reviews of the literature, the benefits of eating fish outweigh risks.[217]

The *omega-3 fatty acids*, *DHA* and *EPA*, are prevalent in the brain, eyes, adrenal glands, and male testes. *DHA* is a primary fat present in the brain, nervous system, and retina of the eye. In fact, the brain is composed largely of fat and DHA is the primary fat in the brain. Omega-3 fatty acids are particularly important for optimal brain and retinal development, maturation of the visual cortex, and motor development in unborn babies. During the third trimester of pregnancy large amounts of the omega-6 fatty acid, AA

---

[211] Br J Psychiatry v.190, p.118, Feb 2007

[212] Biol Psychiatry v.61, No.4, p.551, 2/15/07

[213] Arch Neurol. v. 62, No.12, p.1849, Dec 2005

[214] Prog Neuropsychopharmacol Biol Psychiatry v.31, No.1, p.12, 1/30/07

[215] JAMA v.296, No.15, p.1885, 10/18/06

[216] Lancet v.369, No.9561, p.578, Feb 17, 2007

[217] Harv Health Lett v.32, No.4, p.6, Feb 2007

(arachidonic acid), and the omega-3 fatty acid DHA are required for the increase in growth of neural and vascular systems in a developing baby. Approximately 50 percent of the total fatty acids in the phospholipids of the cerebral cortex (in the brain) and retina consist of the omega-3 fatty acid DHA. Because it has been found that there are diminished levels of DHA in cell membranes during lactation and pregnancy, it is important that pregnant women consume sufficient amounts of omega-3 fatty acids.[218]

Studies have also revealed that people who eat diets containing generous amounts of omega-3 rich fish have a lower risk of autoimmune diseases. Adding fish and other omega-3 rich foods may be beneficial for autoimmune diseases. In addition, omega-3 fatty acids, especially *DHA*, are also being looked at for their potential benefits in mood, memory, learning, brain function, stress response, and even prevention of Alzheimer's disease.

The importance of an omega-3 rich diet cannot be overemphasized.

Omega-6 Fatty Acids: Benefits, Balance, and Transfats

The American population consumes relatively low levels of omega-3 fatty acids compared to omega-6 fatty acids. Today, major food sources of omega-3 essential fatty acids have been exchanged for omega-6 sources to increase the food's shelf life. In addition, the flesh of today's meats and poultry contain more omega-6 fats and are deficient in omega-3 fats due to what they are fed. While the medical community has emphasized the omega-6 linoleic acid oils as a source of polyunsaturated fat, they have not publicized the benefits of the omega-3 polyunsaturated fats. We should consume a diet with a more balanced omega-6 to omega-3 ratio, near four to one, and since omega-6 is far more prevalent in food, we need to emphasize omega-3 rich foods and try to obtain only the highest quality of omega-6-rich food.[219]

It has been reported[220] that human beings started out with a diet consisting of approximately equal amounts of omega-3 and omega-6 essential fatty acids, whereas in Western diets the ratio is 15/1 to 16.7/1. Over the past 100 to 150 years, there has been an increase in the consumption of omega-6 fatty acids because of our increased intake of vegetable oils from corn, sunflower seeds,

---

[218] Science v.278, No.5345, p.1904, 12/12/97

[219] The Journal of Nutrition v.128, No.2, p.427, February 1998

[220] Biomed Pharmacother. v.60, No.9, p.502, Nov 2006

safflower seeds, cottonseed, and soybeans. Studies indicate that a high intake of omega-6 fatty acids can produce negative effects such as increased blood viscosity, vasoconstriction, and decreased bleeding time. On the other hand omega-3 fatty acids have many beneficial effects including lowering the risk or lessening the severity of heart disease, hypertension, Type II diabetes, renal disease, rheumatoid arthritis, and inflammatory and autoimmune diseases, and also may suppress interleukin-1-beta, tumor necrosis factor-alpha, and interleukin-6, as well as the benefits mentioned in the preceding discussion on omega-3 fatty acids.[221]

Researchers report that increasing evidence associates deficiencies or imbalances of omega-3 and omega-6 fatty acids with dyslexia, and found that better word reading was associated with higher total omega-3 concentrations in both dyslexic and control groups. Their results suggested that it is the omega-3/omega-6 balance that is particularly relevant to dyslexia.[222] Two additional studies examining the ratios of omega-6 to omega-3 fatty acids found that increasing dietary omega-3 relative to omega-6 showed favorable results and warranted further investigation in the treatment of prostate cancer[223] and inflammatory bowel disease.[224]

Omega-6 fatty acids are, however, *essential*, therefore required by the body, and have many health benefits. Two rich sources of *omega-6* fatty acids, evening primrose oil and borage oil, which can be found in health food stores, have been studied for their benefits in rheumatologic conditions such as rheumatoid arthritis. In one study it was shown that taking evening primrose oil supplements increases the levels of a certain compound that acts as a competitive inhibitor against formation of the proinflammatory molecules obtained from other omega-6 fats. By blocking the production of proinflammatory molecules when omega-6 fats are consumed, inflammation can actually be suppressed in conditions such as rheumatoid arthritis.[225]

Quality sources of the *omega-6* fatty acids that can be obtained in a health food store include evening primrose oil, borage oil, black currant seed oil, and gooseberry oils. More common healthy sources of *omega-6* fatty acids include raw nuts and seeds, legumes, leafy green vegetables, and grains. Vegetable oils, such as corn, safflower, sunflower, soybean, cottonseed, and

---

[221] American J of Clinical Nutrition v.70, No.3, p.560, Sept 1999; Biomed Pharmacother. v.60, No.9, p.502, Nov 2006

[222] Eur Neuropsychopharmacol v.17, No.2, p.116, 1/15/07

[223] Clin Cancer Res v.12, No.15, p.4662, 8/1/06

[224] Lipids Health Dis. v.5, p.6, 3/20/06

[225] American Journal of Clinical Nutrition v.71, No.1, p.352, January 2000

sesame contain omega-6 fatty acids, but these oils are generally processed, and should be limited as they contain harmful *transfats* as well as contributing to the excess of omega-6 fats in our diets.

Numerous researchers have evaluated the negative effects of **transfats**. *Transfatty acids*, or transfats, are believed to contribute to clogged arteries, heart disease, diabetes, and degenerative diseases. They also lower the good HDL cholesterol while raising the bad LDL cholesterol.[226] Most commercial oils found in grocery stores have been processed using heat and pressure in the presence of a chemical catalyst, which creates transfats. Transfats are named due to how a fat molecule bends at the location of its double bonds. Margarines are produced by hydrogenating oils so that some of their double bonds are changed to single bonds and they become more of a solid at room temperature. Transfats are prevalent in hydrogenated vegetable oils, margarine, artificial cheese, shortening, fried foods, various commercial baked goods including breads, biscuits, cakes, cookies, crackers, corn chips, doughnuts, muffins, pies, potato chips, and rolls. These foods should be limited or avoided. *It is best to choose olive and canola oils instead of grocery store vegetable oils.*

Benefits of Monounsaturated Fatty Acids

Another important group of fats are *monounsaturated fatty acids*, also referred to as the *omega-9 fatty acids*. Contrary to popular belief, low-fat diets appear to be less helpful in the reduction of cardiovascular disease than diets high in monounsaturated fatty acids. High–monounsaturated fatty acid diets lower both blood cholesterol and triacylglycerol (triglycerides) concentrations, but they do not lower HDL (good) cholesterol. In contrast low-fat diets can increase blood triglycerides and decrease HDL (good) cholesterol concentrations, thereby not providing the benefits of diets rich in monounsaturated fatty acid.

It was concluded from a study that a high-monounsaturated diet may be preferable to a low-fat diet because of its more favorable effects on the cardiovascular disease risk profile.[227] In this study the cardiovascular disease risk profile was compared for: (1) the average American diet, (2) a low-fat American Heart Association diet, and (3) high-monounsaturated fat diets rich

---

[226] Science News v.160, No.19, p.300, Nov. 10 2001

[227] American Journal of Clinical Nutrition v. 70, No. 6, 1009, December 1999

in *olive oil, peanut oil,* and *peanuts* and *peanut butter.* The data showed that both the high-monounsaturated fat diets and the low-fat diet lowered total cholesterol and LDL (bad) cholesterol. The low-fat diet, however, raised triacylglycerol (triglycerides) while the high-monounsaturated diets lowered triglycerides. In addition, the low-fat diet lowered HDL (good) cholesterol, while the high monounsaturated diets did not lower HDL (good) cholesterol. Overall, the high monounsaturated-fat diets lowered the risk for cardiovascular disease more than the low-fat diet.

Good sources of monounsaturated fats include olive oil, canola oil, avocados, and nuts such as almonds, pistachios, pecans, cashews, hazelnuts, macadamia nuts, and peanuts. Olive oil, which defines the Mediterranean diet, is associated with positive benefits in cardiovascular disease, lipoprotein profile, blood pressure, glucose metabolism, antithrombotic profile, endothelial function, inflammation, antioxidant properties, age-related cognitive decline, Alzheimer's disease, and healthier aging and increased longevity.[228]

Numerous studies support the finding that diets high in *monounsaturated fats* can lower the risk of cardiovascular disease more than the standard low-fat heart-healthy diets. One study revealed that substituting *almonds* and *almond oil* for other fats in the diet lowered both total cholesterol and low-density lipoprotein (bad) cholesterol. A similar study at the University of Hawaii demonstrated that diets rich in *macadamia nuts* lowered both total blood cholesterol and triglyceride levels, whereas a low-fat diet raised trigyceride levels. A study at the Harvard School of Public Health investigated links between diet and heart disease. This research was part of the Nurses' Health Study of 86,000 women. The data showed that women who consumed an average of at least 5 ounces of nuts a week were only 65% as likely to have suffered coronary heart disease, including fatal heart attacks, as those women who rarely ate nuts.[229] A review of five studies on the benefits of walnuts consistently demonstrated walnuts as part of a heart-healthy diet, lower blood cholesterol concentrations. These results were supported by several large additional studies demonstrating a dose response-related association between a reduced risk of coronary heart disease and the frequent daily consumption of small amounts of nuts, including walnuts.[230] Data from among 21,454 male participants enrolled in the US Physicians' Health Study, in which

---

[228] Eur J Clin Invest v.35, No.7, p421, Jul 2005

[229] Science News v.154, No.21, p.328, 11/21/98

[230] J Nutr. v.132, No.5, p.1062-1101, May 2002

participants were followed up for an average of 17 years, revealed that dietary nut intake was associated with a significantly reduced risk of sudden cardiac death after controlling for known cardiac risk factors and other dietary habits.[231]

Nuts are not only high in monounsaturated and polyunsaturated fatty acids, but they appear to contain other bioactive molecules that possess cardio-protective effects. These bioactive molecules may include plant proteins, dietary fiber, micronutrients such as copper and magnesium, plant sterols, and phytochemicals. More specifically, researchers believe that there are molecules in nuts that have cholesterol-lowering effects in addition to the cholesterol-lowering effects of the fatty acids.[232] In addition to their monounsaturated fatty acid content, nuts are also good sources of protein, antioxidants, calcium, magnesium, boron, vitamin-E, zinc, selenium, essential fatty acids, biotin, B-vitamins, and fiber. After cereals, nuts are the vegetable foods that are richest in fiber, which may partly explain their benefit on the lipid profile and cardiovascular health.[233]

Our diets should be rich in mono-unsaturated fats such as olive oil, canola oil, and nuts.

Protein

Research indicates that diets higher in protein boost blood levels of a hormone recently found to curb appetite.[234] *Proteins* are made up of 22 amino acids of which 9 are essential and must be obtained from our food. Proteins comprise about fifty percent of our dry weight, which means if the water in our bodies was removed, we would consist of about fifty percent protein.[235] In our living 'wet-weight' form, our bodies are primarily comprised of about 60% water, 20% fat, and 20% protein, carbohydrates, bone minerals, and other minerals and vitamins.[236] If we want our bodies to be healthy, energetic, and function properly, we must consume the essential amino acids that make up protein foods. Proteins, or their amino acid components, can be obtained from various foods such as fish, tofu, tempeh,

---

[231] Arch Intern Med. v.162, No.12, p.1382, 6/24/02

[232] American Journal of Clinical Nutrition v.70, No.3, p.504, Sept 1999

[233] Br J Nutr. v.96 Suppl 2, p.45, Nov 2006

[234] Cell Metabolism September 2006/ Science News v.170, No.11, p.173, 9/9/06

[235] Your Body Knows Best, Ann Louise Gittleman, Pocket, 1997 p.81

[236] Nutrition: Concepts and Controversy, Hamilon, 1985, p.15

soybeans, nuts, seeds, beans, legumes, wheat germ, sprouted beans and grains, vegetables, protein drinks, organic yogurt and other animal protein such as organic cottage cheese, eggs, and meat. (If you eat dairy, meat, or poultry, use only organic to avoid hormones, antibiotics, chemicals, or drugs from animals fed these chemicals as well as feed containing diseased or same-species meat.)

Proteins are essential for the functioning of our bodies and are generally involved in production, growth, repair and maintenance of cells, tissues, hormones, enzymes, muscles, skin, organs, blood, blood cells, connective tissue, bones, neurotransmitters, the immune system, antibodies, hair, nails, and antioxidants, as well as wound healing, brain function, and stabilizing blood sugar. More specifically, proteins are involved in building muscle tissue, increasing metabolism, growth and repair of cells and tissues, hormone production, enzyme production, neurotransmitter production, function of the immune system, antibody production, fluid balance, wound healing, antioxidant activity, brain function, stabilizing of blood sugar, hair and nail growth, growth-hormone production, production of the pancreatic hormone *glucagon,* and maintenance of muscles, skin, organs, blood, blood cells, connective tissue, bones, and the nervous system.

Researchers have found that diets containing sufficient amounts of protein are important to the health of our hearts. The association between dietary protein intake and incidence of heart disease was examined in a group of 80,082 women in the Nurse's Health Study who had no previous diagnosis of heart disease, stroke, cancer, hypercholesterolemia, or diabetes. Researchers documented 939 major instances of heart disease during 14 years of follow-up. It was found that after age, smoking, total calorie intake, percentages of calorie from specific types of fat, and other heart disease risk factors were controlled for, higher protein intakes were associated with a lower risk of heart disease. Nurses consuming approximately 24 percent of their calories from protein had only about three-quarters of the *heart disease* risk found in the women who obtained approximately 15 percent of their calories from protein. Both animal and vegetable proteins contributed to the lower risk. This inverse association was similar for women eating low- or high-fat diets. The findings of this study suggest that replacing some carbohydrates with protein may be associated with a lower risk of heart disease.[237]

---

[237] American J of Clinical Nutrition v.70, No.2, p.221, Aug 1999; Science News v.156, No.6, p.86, 8/7/99

In addition, a further study was done in which men and women at risk for heart disease were switched between diets having low and high amounts of protein. Results showed that during high-protein eating periods the participants' blood concentrations of triglycerides and low-density lipoproteins (bad cholesterol) fell, while high-density lipoprotein (good cholesterol) rose. These changes during the high-protein phase are believed to reduce heart-disease risk.[238] Eating healthy fats, such as olive oil, fish oil, and nuts, along with the proper amount of dietary protein, can benefit our long-term health.

In a recent study on the association between high- and low-carbohydrate diets and the risk of coronary heart disease, it was reported that a diet rich in high glycemic index foods (carbohydrates that raise blood sugar quickly) was strongly associated with an increased risk of coronary heart disease. These researchers also found that diets lower in carbohydrates and higher in protein and fat do not increase the risk of coronary heart disease (as once thought), and *when dietary protein and fat is from vegetable sources*, these diets can reduce the risk of coronary heart disease.[239] Epidemiologic studies have shown a significant relationship between increased protein intake and lower risk of hypertension and coronary heart disease. Evidence from clinical trials also indicates that higher-protein diets improve blood lipids and increase short-term weight loss.[240] A study comparing high protein to high carbohydrate diets showed that a diet with higher protein and lower carbohydrates combined with exercise improved body composition during weight loss.[241]

Because of the critical functions of proteins in our body, it is important to supply ourselves with adequate protein from the foods we eat. In view of the fact that experts disagree on the actual percentage of protein in the diet that is most healthy, it is a good idea to talk to your doctor. If you derive part of your protein from eating meat or poultry, it is important to eat grain-fed, organically-raised meats. Also, it is important to avoid raw or undercooked meats, raw or undercooked fish, and raw or undercooked eggs to protect yourself from bacteria, viruses, or parasites that may be present in these raw foods.

---

[238] Science News v.156, No.6, p.86, 8/7/99

[239] N. Engl. J. Med. v..355, No.19, p1991, 11/9/06

[240] Journal of Clinical Nutrition v.82, No.1, p.242, July 2005

[241] J. Nutr. v.135, p.1903, August 2005

If You Are Vegetarian or Nearly Vegetarian

Emphasizing plant foods in your diet is healthy as a general practice. In fact, it has been shown that a high consumption of plant-based foods such as fruit and vegetables, nuts, and whole grains is associated with a significantly lower risk of coronary artery disease and stroke.[242] A recent review[243] of vegetarians and non-vegetarians revealed that vegetarians tend to weigh less than non-vegetarians and have a lower incidence of certain diseases associated with overweight and obese individuals, such as heart disease, diabetes, high blood pressure, and certain cancers.

If you do not eat much meat, and have a mostly vegetarian diet, you may be somewhat deficient in *vitamin B12* as well as *zinc* and should talk to your doctor about taking B12 and zinc supplements along with a good multi-vitamin/mineral supplement. Zinc is important for functioning of the immune and reproductive systems and in the synthesis and function of adrenal cortical hormones and insulin. Zinc is found in oysters, crab, beef, poultry, eggs, pumpkin seeds, almonds, cashews, sea vegetables, and wheat germ. A problem with many vegetarian sources of zinc is that they also have high amounts of copper, which acts as an antagonist to zinc. Foods rich in copper include whole grains, nuts, soy products, organ meats, and shellfish. Vegetarians usually eat generous amounts of grains, soy, and nuts, and therefore are more likely to get abundant amounts of copper. The RDA for copper is 2 milligrams and for zinc 15 milligrams, which means the proper balance of zinc to copper in the body is approximately 8 to 1. If you are vegetarian and consume excessive copper as compared to zinc, it may make sense to balance high copper containing foods with zinc containing foods and/or zinc supplements. You should talk with your doctor about supplements.

Vitamin B12, or *Cobalamin*, is found in the most sufficient amounts in animal products and should be supplemented in vegetarian diets. Vitamin B12 is involved in the formation and regeneration of red blood cells, maintenance of the nervous system, growth in children, energy production, calcium absorption, and metabolism of carbohydrates, fats and protein. It has been reported that vitamin B12 deficiency was shown to occur in children on macrobiotic or vegan diets. Furthermore, moderate consumption of animal products was not sufficient to restore normal cobalamin status in

---

[242] American Journal of Clinical Nutrition v.78, No.3, p.544, September 2003

[243] Nutrition Reviews v.64, No.4, p.175, April 2006

patients with inadequate cobalamin intake during their early years of life.[244] According to the U. S. Food and Drug Administration, about 10 to 20 percent of elderly people are diagnosed as having low vitamin B12 levels.[245] If your diet is low in animal products, talk to your doctor about whether you should supplement B12 and, if so, how much.

Sugars and Carbohydrates

Research studies have found that people who eat a diet high in *sugars* and low-fiber *carbohydrates* are more likely to become diabetic than those who eat less refined foods.[246] In fact, sugar is probably one of the most dangerous natural foods that we eat in large quantities. Unfortunately, Americans consume somewhere in the neighborhood of 150 pounds of sugar per person per year.[247] There has been a dramatic increase in sugar consumption from the early 1800's, when Americans consumed 12 pounds per person per year, through the early 1900's, when Americans consumed 65 to 95 pounds per person per year, to the present 150 pounds per person per year.[248] This translates to approximately 0.41 pounds or approaching a half of a pound of sugar per day! Recent increases in consumption of added sugars in the U.S. can increase the overall caloric intake and significantly reduce intake of vital nutrients. As was evident in a study of low-income households, added sugars should be discouraged as they adversely affect diet quality and decrease dietary nutrients including protein, iron, and vitamins A, C, B6 and B12.[249]

Low-fat, low-protein, high-carbohydrate diets became popular in the U.S. because they have been thought to be helpful in reducing heart disease and some cancers. It turns out that plant-based diets that are not low-fat, but are rich in unsaturated fatty acids and include nuts, seeds, fish, olive oil, and oils from grains, nuts, seeds, and fish, do not increase but actually reduce the risk of heart disease. In addition, for people with insulin resistance (discussed below), higher healthy-fat diets help protect against the heart disease risk factors. Furthermore, people on low-fat diets actually produce more fatty acid in their bodies, which may indicate that diets very low in all types of fat

---

[244] American Journal of Clinical Nutrition v.69, No.4, 664, April 1999

[245] http://vm.cfsan.fda.gov/~dms/wh-folic.html

[246] JAMA v.277, No.6, p.472, 1997

[247] Science News v.154, No.11, p.171, 9/12/98

[248] Get The Sugar Out, Ann Louise Gittleman, Three Rivers Press, 1996, p. xiii

[249] Journal of Nutrition v.137, No.2, p.453, Feb 2007

could adversely affect the overall risk for heart disease.[250] In fact, as mentioned in the above section, *Fats*, diets rich in monounsaturated fats found in nuts, olive oil, and canola oil, as well as omega-3 fatty acids found in flaxseed oil, fish, and fish oil, are believed to lower the risk of heart disease more than low-fat, high-carbohydrate diets. In a recent study on the association between high- and low-carbohydrate diets and the risk of coronary heart disease, it was reported that a diet rich in high glycemic index foods (carbohydrates that raise blood sugar quickly) was strongly associated with an increased risk of coronary heart disease.[251]

The over-consumption of carbohydrates is implicated in the proliferation of adult-onset *diabetes*, a progressive, serious illness with complications such as kidney failure, heart disease, stroke, blindness, nerve damage, circulatory problems, wound healing problems often resulting in amputations, male impotence, and other debilitating health problems. Adult-onset diabetes can develop when the insulin secreted into the bloodstream is insufficient or is unable to effectively balance blood sugar levels and store the blood sugar glucose in the muscles. Other health problems that may be associated with the over consumption of carbohydrates include increased triglyceride levels, hypoglycemia, insulin resistance, and heart disease.

One of the potentially harmful effects of continuously eating excessive amounts of sugar and carbohydrates is that sugar is continually dumped into the bloodstream, followed by a counteracting insulin discharge. Some researchers believe this constant cycle can eventually lead to *insulin resistance* as well as have a negative impact on people who are already insulin resistant. In a person with *insulin resistance,* the normal amount of secreted insulin does not sufficiently lower the blood sugar levels, which causes the pancreas to release excessive amounts of insulin until the blood sugar is normalized. Insulin resistance is not only thought to be a precursor of adult-onset diabetes, but also the buildup of insulin in the bloodstream is believed to be connected to an increase in heart-attack risk. Researchers have found that the buildup of insulin in the blood may prevent the body from breaking down blood clots efficiently contributing to heart-attack risk.[252]

A further consequence of ingesting too many carbohydrates is that it aggravates the problems associated with *Syndrome X.* Syndrome X (first

---

[250] American Journal of Clinical Nutrition v.70, No.3, 512, September 1999

[251] N. Engl. J. Med. v..355, No.19, p.1991, 11/91/06

[252] Science News v.157, No.5, p77, 1/29/00 / JAMA v.283, p.221, 1/12/00

described by Dr. Gerald Reaven of Stanford University) is associated with an increased risk for heart disease. It is believed that Syndrome X is caused by both genetic predisposition and lifestyle, and is defined as a group of risk factors that represent a cause of coronary heart disease. Syndrome X is seen in people who are insulin resistant and involves the body's inability to dispose of glucose in the blood by moving it into muscle and fat cells. Problems associated with Syndrome X include a high insulin level, high triglycerides, low HDL (good) cholesterol, high blood pressure, some degree of glucose intolerance, smaller and denser LDL (bad) cholesterol particles, an increase in the accumulation of triglyceride-rich lipoproteins in the blood, increased tendency of the blood to form clots, and a high plasminogen activator-1 indicating a reduced ability to break up blood clots, which increases heart attack risk. The most common sign of Syndrome X is a high insulin level.[253]

After a healthy person eats, glucose rises in the blood and stimulates the pancreas to secrete insulin. The insulin attaches to the insulin receptors on cell surfaces and enables glucose to enter muscle and fat cells. After an *insulin-resistant* person eats, the pancreas secretes sufficient insulin but the body is resistant to it. The pancreas compensates by secreting more and more insulin to control blood glucose levels. High insulin levels and insulin resistance can lead to symptoms of Syndrome X as well as to Type II diabetes. With *diabetes*, the body secretes more and more insulin, which nevertheless is insufficient and unable to effectively balance blood sugar levels and store glucose (sugar) in the muscles cells, resulting in a rise in blood glucose levels.

There is also a connection between chronically high insulin levels in the blood and Alzheimer's disease. Chronically high insulin levels in the blood appear to cause the accumulation of beta-amyloid protein in the brain (a characteristic of Alzheimer's disease) and therefore may play a role in Alzheimer's disease. Consistent with this finding is that people with Type II diabetes, which is characterized by high levels of insulin circulating in the blood, have an increased risk of Alzheimer's disease. Several studies have shown that people with Type II diabetes have twice the risk of developing the disease as non-diabetics.[254] Whether the increase in Alzheimer's disease is due to high blood insulin or other factors related to diabetes has not been proven as yet, but avoiding diabetes (as well as insulin resistance) will

---

[253] Nutrition Action Health Letter v.27, No.2, March 2000

[254] Science v.301, No.5629, p.40, 7/4/03

certainly reduce the significant diabetes-related risk factor for Alzheimer's disease.

Researchers believe that losing weight, restricting carbohydrates, limiting foods that rapidly release sugar into the bloodstream (high-glycemic index foods), and substituting monounsaturated and polyunsaturated fats into the diet can help people with insulin resistance.[255]

When any food containing carbohydrates is eaten, the carbohydrates are digested and broken down to provide blood sugar requirements. Simple sugars and processed carbohydrates enter the bloodstream quickly while complex carbohydrates enter more gradually. It is not necessary to eat pure sugar or processed carbohydrates to supply blood sugar. In fact, at a stable blood sugar level, the human bloodstream should only contain about two teaspoons of glucose.[256] When foods high in sugars and processed carbohydrates are ingested, sugar is rapidly released into the bloodstream. This causes the body to react by secreting *insulin* from the pancreas into the bloodstream to bring down the blood sugar to a healthy level. Insulin facilitates the storage of a limited amount of sugar in the liver and muscles as glycogen for energy, and the remaining sugar is stored as body fat in fat tissues. If a person hasn't eaten for a while, their blood sugar will eventually fall. When blood sugar falls, the pancreas secretes the hormone glucagon, which converts glycogen (a stored form of sugar) back into glucose in order to restore the proper equilibrium blood sugar level.

Studies have shown that diets based on foods that release sugar into the bloodstream more slowly (low-glycemic index foods) improved serum triglyceride levels, total cholesterol levels, and the ratio of LDLs to HDLs.[257] In addition, a study found that colon cancer patients were twice as likely as other people to regularly eat high-glycemic index foods, which release sugar rapidly and put a high insulin demand on the body.[258] (See page 147 for a listing of high- and low-glycemic index foods.)

It has been reported[259] that the long-term consumption of foods that quickly digest into simple sugars may cause the body to produce excess insulin and abdominal fat. In an Australian research study, rats were fed diets consisting

---

[255] Science News v.157, No.15, p. 236, 4/8/00

[256] The 40/30/30 Phenomenon, Ann Louise Gittleman, Keats Publishing 1999 p.18

[257] Science News v.157, No.15, p. 236, 4/8/00

[258] Science News v.157, No.19, p.298, 5/6/00

[259] Science News v.159, No.7 p.111, 2/17/01

of 20 percent protein, 35 percent fat, and 45 percent carbohydrates (consisting of sugars and starch), with half of the animals receiving low-glycemic index carbohydrates that digest more slowly and half receiving high-glycemic index carbohydrates, which digest rapidly releasing sugar more quickly into the blood.[260] Results from the study demonstrated that while both groups of rats weighed about the same, the high-glycemic index fed rats had more abdominal fat and showed blood concentrations of insulin that peaked more quickly after a meal and remained high longer than low-glycemic index fed rats. The researchers believe that over-secretion of insulin produced the extra fat in the high-glycemic index animals. In addition, these rats produced excessive insulin in response to every sugar and starch they consumed not just high-glycemic index carbohydrates.

While the hypothesis that a low-fat diet can reduce breast cancer risk has existed for decades, in a controlled intervention trial of postmenopausal women it was found that a low-fat diet did not result in a statistically significant reduction in invasive breast cancer risk over an 8.1-year average follow-up period.[261] Another study focused on an area of breast cancer research involving the impact of reproductive steroid hormones (serum estradiol) on breast cancer development and recurrence. These hormones may have adverse affects on breast tissue. Results from this study indicated that a high-fiber, low-fat diet may be helpful in reducing blood levels of these reproductive steroid hormones in women diagnosed with breast cancer. Increased fiber intake was also independently related to the reduction in serum estradiol concentration.[262] The take-home message from these studies is that while a low fat diet has not been shown to reduce breast cancer risk, having a lot of fiber in your diet offers a number of benefits including reducing levels of certain potentially harmful hormones. Achieving and maintaining a healthy weight and eating nutritiously will help you stay healthy and recover from diseases including breast cancer.

A study evaluating weight and heart health by comparing a low-carbohydrate diet versus a low-fat, low-cholesterol diet found that a greater proportion of the low-carbohydrate diet group were able to remain on their diets and complete the study (76% vs. 57%). At 24 weeks, weight loss was greater in the low-carbohydrate diet group than in the low-fat diet group. Compared with recipients of the low-fat diet, recipients of the low-carbohydrate diet

[260] Science News v.157, No.15, p.236, 4/8/00

[261] JAMA v.295, No.6, p.629, 2/8/06

[262] J Clin Oncol. v.22, No.12, p.2379, 6/15/04

had greater decreases in serum triglyceride levels and greater increases in high-density lipoprotein (good) cholesterol levels. Changes in low-density lipoprotein cholesterol level did not differ statistically between the diets.[263] Another study comparing the effects of a moderate-fat diet (30% calories from fat) versus a low-fat one (20% calories from fat) found the moderate-fat diet was more successful after 14 months in reducing weight, waist circumference, and other cardiovascular risk factors including LDL (bad) cholesterol, TAG, total cholesterol, and systolic blood pressure. The researchers concluded that a moderate-fat calorie-restricted diet in the long term might have more beneficial effects on weight maintenance and cardiovascular risk factors than a low-fat diet.[264] The majority of studies I have read on dietary fat seem to reveal that having healthy fats in your diet is a benefit.

What Are Carbohydrates and Carbohydrate Foods?

Carbohydrates provide sugar that is burned in the muscles and brain for energy. Carbohydrates can be simple or complex. Simple carbohydrates, or sugars, consist of one or two sugar molecules, and include table sugar, brown sugar, honey, corn syrup, glucose (dextrose), sucrose, barley malt, maltodextrin, sucrose, fructose in fruits, and lactose in milk and milk products. Simple sugars are absorbed quickly into the bloodstream and raise blood sugar rapidly.

Complex carbohydrates are made up of chains of simple sugars and are found in a variety of foods such as grains, vegetables, beans, legumes, and starches. *Starches* are a family of carbohydrates that consist of linked glucose molecules. Complex carbohydrates generally absorb more slowly providing a steadier blood sugar rise. Some complex carbohydrates found in foods such as carrots, potatoes, white rice, and corn, however, have a high *glycemic index* and break down quickly causing a rapid increase in blood sugar. The *glycemic index* is a measure of how fast carbohydrates are absorbed into the bloodstream and raise the blood sugar level. Processed complex carbohydrates have been refined to the point that they behave more like simple carbohydrates and break down quickly causing a rapid increase in blood sugar levels. Processed carbohydrates include pasta, white flour, white rice, breads, muffins, bagels, pastries, and most commercial cereals.

---

[263] Ann Intern Med. v.140, No.10, p.769, 5/18/04

[264] Br J Nutr. v.97, No.2, p.399, Feb 2007

The carbohydrates we eat should be primarily complex and have a low glycemic index so that they break down into glucose in the bloodstream more slowly. A glycemic index above 70 percent represents foods that absorb quickly and raise the blood sugar rapidly; a glycemic index under 40 percent represents foods that absorb slowly and raise the blood sugar more slowly; and a glycemic index between 40 and 70 represent foods that absorb and raise blood sugar moderately. The following are examples of carbohydrate containing foods having high, moderate, and low *glycemic indexes*:[265]

Carbohydrate-rich foods with high glycemic index (70 to 100):

Refined breakfast cereals, sugar, honey, white bread, most crackers, graham crackers, white rice, rolled oats, oat bran, oatmeal cookies, whole-wheat bread, corn chips, white bagels, croissants, pretzels, carrots, baked potatoes, cooked potatoes, jams, bananas, pineapples, and raisins.

Carbohydrate-rich foods with moderate glycemic index (40 to 70):

Macaroni, spaghetti, pasta, rye, bulgur, wheat kernels, barley, whole-grain pumpernickel, wheat grain, barley grain, cracked wheat, cracked wheat bread, whole grain breakfast cereals, wild rice, brown rice, peas, navy beans, lima beans, pinto beans, green beans, corn, popcorn, yams, grapes, oranges, apricots, kiwi, and strawberries.

Carbohydrate-containing foods with low glycemic index (0 to 40):

Peanuts, nuts, soybeans, green vegetables, kidney beans, lentils, chickpeas (garbanzos), tomatoes, tomato soup, milk, plain yogurt, grapefruit, cherries, apples, pears, plums, and peaches.

Eating proteins, fats, and low-glycemic index foods along with a high-glycemic index foods can help the high-glycemic index food to absorb more slowly as they mix together. Plant-based foods that are very low in sugar and do not raise blood sugar rapidly include olives, olive oil, canola oil, lettuce, cucumbers, radishes, peppers, celery, alfalfa sprouts, asparagus, green beans, cabbage, cauliflower, eggplant, scallions, onions, leeks, spinach, squash, pumpkin, snow peas, broccoli, kale, avocados, tomatoes, water chestnuts, artichoke hearts, Brussels sprouts, and bean sprouts. Plant-based foods that have a low glycemic index are also generally high in fiber, which provides a sense of fullness and is beneficial for elimination. If you are not getting

---

[265] Science News v.157, No.15, p. 236, 4/8/00; American Journal of Clinical Nutrition v.76, No.1, p.5-56, 2002

enough fiber, you may want to ask your doctor about adding a psyllium husk product to your diet.

In your daily diet, it is best to limit sugars and processed carbohydrates and to eat foods with a low glycemic index and high fiber content. You will ingest more than enough sugar in fruits, vegetables, and non-processed complex carbohydrates – you don't need extra. Try to eat primarily healthy complex carbohydrates, such as unprocessed whole grains, beans and legumes.

You may be regularly ingesting a lot of sugar and wonder if you will be able to limit it in the future. Consider that many of our tastes in foods developed as habits and can be changed by developing new habits of not eating a certain food or transferring to a healthy food. Don't add sugar to foods and drinks. Don't keep sweets around your home. Sweeten foods with fruit, dried fruit, or, if necessary, a limited amount of honey. Also, watch out for so-called "low-fat" foods as they are often saturated with excess sugar. Low-fat foods often have close to as many calories as their "normal-fat" counterparts, along with other undesirable additives such as sugar. If you must add a small amount of sweetener to your coffee, tea, or whole grain cereal, use a limited amount of honey rather than sugar. Unlike sugar, honey actually has beneficial properties. Honey contains significant quantities of antioxidants, and has also been shown to slow the oxidation of fats in foods.[266] But try to wean yourself off sugar. Finally, keep artificial sweeteners out of your body – their potential side effects may be worse than the sugar they replace.

Overall, obtaining good nutrition is serious and challenging, and depends on you, but can be fun and tasty if you're creative.

A Word About Food Allergies and Intolerance[267]

True *food allergies* affect an estimated 2 percent of adults and 2 to 8 percent of children. *Food intolerance* is much more common than food allergies, but may produce symptoms similar to food allergies, such as abdominal cramping. The difference between an allergy and an intolerance is how the body handles the offending food. In an allergy the immune system reacts to an allergen, usually a protein, in the offending food, whereas an intolerance

---

[266] Science News v.154, No.11, p.171, 9/12/98

[267] U.S. Food and Drug Administration FDA Consumer May 1994; Updated Dec. 2004: http://vm.cfsan.fda.gov/~dms/wh-alrg1.html,; http://www.wellweb.com/nutri/food_allergies_rare_but_risky.htm; http://www.aaaai.org/patients/publicedmat/tips/foodallergy.stm

involves the body's inability to adequately digest some component of the food. People with a food intolerance can often eat some of the offending food without experiencing symptoms.

Foods that commonly cause an allergic reaction include cow's milk, eggs, wheat, soy foods, tree nuts, fish, shellfish, and peanuts. Adverse or allergic reactions also can come from citrus fruits, corn, refined sugar, artificial food coloring, food additives and preservatives, tomatoes, eggplant, chocolate, onions, and strawberries. Common allergic reactions to foods include swelling in the mouth, lips or tongue; itching lips; wheezing or breathing problems; hives; rashes; stomach cramps; vomiting; diarrhea; and in some cases serious illness or even death. The most serious reaction to a food allergy is anaphylaxis, also known as anaphylactic shock, which is a severe allergic reaction involving a number of parts of the body simultaneously. Signs of a severe reaction include difficulty breathing, feeling of impending doom, swelling of the mouth and throat, a drop in blood pressure, and loss of consciousness. If you see signs of a severe allergic reaction, get medical help immediately.

Food additives such as aspartame, monosodium glutamate (MSG), sulfur-based preservatives (sulfites), and tartrazine, also known as FD&C Yellow No. 5 can also cause adverse reactions. Aspartame, or Nutrasweet, should be avoided by people with the disease phenylketonuria, or those with advanced liver disease, as well as pregnant women with hyperphenylalanine (high levels of phenylalanine in the blood). MSG has been associated with headaches, tightness in the chest, and nervousness, and is being studied by the FDA. The food color, FD&C Yellow No. 5 (listed as tartrazine on medicine labels), is associated with itching or hives in sensitive people. Sulfur-based food additives (sulfites) are used to prevent or reduce discoloration in fruits and vegetables, and to inhibit the growth of microorganisms in fermented foods, such as wine, and can cause mild to life-threatening reactions that resemble food allergens. The FDA has ruled that the addition of aspartame, MSG, FD&C Yellow No. 5, and sulfur-based additives to a product must be declared on the label.

Appendix 2:

BODY MASS INDEX (BMI)

A transition is underway in the United States to identify and classify overweight and obese adults using body mass index, or BMI. As BMI value increases, the risk for some diseases increases. BMI is calculated using weight and height. To obtain your BMI you can use the chart below. If your height or weight isn't listed, or you want to compute your exact BMI value, multiply your weight (in pounds) by 703 and then divide it by your height (in inches) squared, or:

$$\text{BMI} = [(\text{Your weight in pounds}) \times (703)] \div [(\text{Your height in inches})^2]$$
$$= [(\text{Your weight in pounds}) \times (703)] \div [(\text{Your height in inches}) \times (\text{Your height in inches})]$$

		19	20	21	22	23	24	25	26	27	28	29	30	35	40
				W E I G H T				(p o u n d s)							
	4'10"	91	96	100	105	110	115	119	124	129	134	138	143	167	191
	4'11"	94	99	104	109	114	119	124	128	133	138	143	148	173	198
	5'0"	97	102	107	112	118	123	128	133	138	143	148	153	179	204
H	5'1"	100	106	111	116	122	127	132	137	143	148	153	158	185	211
	5'2"	104	109	115	120	126	131	136	142	147	153	158	164	191	218
E	5'3"	107	113	118	124	130	135	141	146	152	158	163	169	197	225
	5'4"	110	116	122	128	134	140	145	151	157	163	169	174	204	232
I	5'5"	114	120	126	132	138	144	150	156	162	168	174	180	210	240
	5'6"	118	124	130	136	142	148	155	161	167	173	179	186	216	247
G	5'7"	121	127	134	140	146	153	159	166	172	178	185	191	223	255
	5'8"	125	131	138	144	151	158	164	171	177	184	190	197	230	262
H	5'9"	128	135	142	149	155	162	169	176	182	189	196	203	236	270
	5'10"	132	139	146	153	160	167	174	181	188	195	202	207	243	278
T	5'11"	136	143	150	157	165	172	179	186	193	200	208	215	250	286
	6'0"	140	147	154	162	169	177	184	191	199	206	213	221	258	294
	6'1"	144	151	159	166	174	182	189	197	204	212	219	227	265	302
	6'2"	148	155	163	171	179	186	194	202	210	218	225	233	272	311
	6'3"	152	160	168	176	184	192	200	208	216	224	232	240	279	319
	6'4"	156	164	172	180	189	197	205	213	221	230	238	246	287	328
								O V E R W E I G H T					O B E S E		

Caption above table: **B O D Y   M A S S   I N D E X   (B M I)**

http://www.consumer.gov/weightloss/bmi.htm

Note that two people can have the same BMI, but a different percent body fat. For example, a muscular athlete with a low percent body fat may have the same BMI as a person with a higher percent body fat. Similarly, for the same BMI value, women are more likely to have a higher percent body fat than men. While BMI can be valuable for assessing obesity and disease risk, it should be used in conjunction with other risk factors, such as the measure of waist circumference.

Index

How To Begin

You can work your way into *The 3:00 PM Secret* lifestyle by progressing through the three steps described below. You can spend up to several weeks in each of the first two steps before moving on to the final step.

STEP 1

1. You must (once and for all) **decide** whether you truly want to spend the rest of your life in your ideal body.

2. Stop eating by 5:00 PM five days a week and shift most of the calories you eat earlier into the day; the other two days are *Free days*.

3. Eat at least *two* servings of fruit and *three* servings of vegetables each day. Drink plenty of water. Begin cutting back on high calorie, low nutrition foods.

4. Begin learning the exercises by doing one or two repetitions of each exercise six days per week. Alternate Upper Body Exercises with Lower Body Exercises every other day. As an alternative to weight-lifting you can use a Nordic Trac, rowing machine, or other resistance-providing equipment.

5. Imagine you have twenty million dollars in the bank and never have to work again...think about how you would spend your time for the rest of your life. What dreams have you been neglecting?

STEP 2

1. Think about what your ideal body looks like.

2. Stop eating by 4:30 PM five days a week for one or two weeks; the other two days are *Free days*. Then stop eating by 4:00 PM five days a week for one or two weeks; the other two days are *Free days*.

3. Focus on nutrition so you don't crave unnecessary calories while your body tries to get the nutrients it needs.
   (a) Eat at least two servings of fruit and at least three servings of vegetables every day.

(b) Consume omega-3 fatty acids from fatty and cold-water fish, fish oil or omega-3 supplements, flaxseed oil, etc.

(c) Begin replacing butter and hydrogenated oils with olive or canola oil.

(d) Begin to limit intake of sugars and processed carbohydrates.

(e) Drink plenty of water and avoid soft drinks and sugary drinks.

(f) Eliminate one trigger food from your house on 3:00 PM days.

(g) Continue to cut back on high calorie, low nutrition foods.

4. Continue getting used to the exercises by doing 4 or 5 repetitions of each exercise six days per week. Alternate Upper Body Exercises with Lower Body Exercises every other day. You may also use resistance-providing equipment.

5. Go to bed (lights out) fifteen to thirty minutes earlier than normal.

6. Spend some time investigating different subjects, activities, or possible vocations that interest you to discover what really captivates you and holds your attention. What dreams have you forgotten?

STEP 3: This is a summary of *The 3:00 PM Secret,* which can be personalized and followed indefinitely.

1. You have made the decision to control your weight and spend the rest of your life in your ideal body. You are on your journey to discover what truly fascinates you and would bring adventure and true meaning into your life. Continue to investigate what really captivates your imagination and how you can incorporate whatever that is into your life. What dreams have you not allowed yourself to consider?

2. Stop eating by 3:30 PM five days a week for one or two weeks; the other two days are Free days. Then stop eating by 3:00 PM five days a week, and you are now in the *rhythm* of *3:00 PM days* and *Free days*. It is recommended that you begin with an eating rhythm of five *3:00 PM days* and two *Free days* each week. If after several weeks, you do not begin to feel your clothes getting looser and experience some weight loss, then you can cut back on what you are consuming on *3:00 PM days*, especially empty calories, or you may want to increase the number of *3:00 PM days* to six days per week and eat fairly lightly in the evening on the seventh day. *Free days* are most useful for social dinners rather than an excuse to overeat. It is best to eat early in the day so you can burn up that food for energy during the day and early evening when you need it.

3. Continue to focus on nutrition.
   (a) Eat 3 to 5 servings of vegetables and 2 to 4 servings of fruit daily.
   (b) Consume omega-3 fatty acids regularly in the form of fatty and cold-water fish, fish oil or omega-3 supplements, flaxseed oil, etc.
   (c) Replace butter and hydrogenated oils with monounsaturated fatty-acid rich olive oil and canola oil.
   (d) Limit sugars, processed carbohydrates, and high-glycemic index carbohydrates.
   (e) Avoid or strictly limit *transfat*-containing foods such as fried foods, margarine, most convenience foods, cookies, pastries, prepared snacks, doughnuts, and hydrogenated vegetable oils.
   (f) Consume sufficient protein.
   (g) Choose *whole-food complex carbohydrates* such as beans, legumes, brown or wild rice, and unprocessed whole grains.
   (h) Drink plenty of water and avoid soft drinks and sugary drinks.
   (i) Take supplements recommended by your doctor.
   (j) Eliminate trigger foods from your house on *3:00 PM days*.
   (k) Avoid or strictly limit high calorie, low nutrition foods.

4. Do the quick, easy, convenient *ten-minute daily workout.* Do one 12-repetition set of each exercise six days per week. Alternate Upper Body Exercises with Lower Body Exercises every other day. You can increase repetitions and weight over time as you feel able. As an alternative to weight lifting you can use a Nordic Trac, rowing machine, or similar resistance-providing equipment.

5. Get 7 to 8 hours of *sleep* so you don't eat for energy because you are tired.

A Note On Habits

People who are able to control their weight are not necessarily more disciplined or smarter, but instead they have developed good habits that have become part of their daily life. The fact that habits are difficult to break can be a blessing in disguise, because once you make good ones and they become ingrained, you will be able to keep them. So, how do you successfully change your habits? My suggestion is *very slowly*. Work through the three-step staging process described above until you are comfortably following *The 3:00 PM Secret*, the 10-minute workout, the ten tips for good nutrition, getting adequate sleep, and focusing on making your life more exciting and meaningful, and beginning to *live your dreams*.

For me, a paramount habit within *The 3:00 PM Secret* that has enabled me to achieve and maintain my desired weigh is to eliminate the habit of eating a meal at night and, in so doing, develop the habit of not eating at night unless I have a special social occasion. Instead of working all day and eating a substantial dinner, I eat breakfast and lunch and have a cup of soymilk or something similar, if needed, at night. Many years ago I would have thought that not eating at night would be an extreme form of torture...but now it is normal. In fact, having my nights free without the burden of preparing, eating, and cleaning up is downright liberating. On top of that, when I do have a meal at night, I feel overfull and don't sleep well.

We do, with some regularity, change our lifestyle and habits throughout our lives, and eventually become comfortable with each new habit that is programmed into our lives. Once you change your habits, you will find what seemed comfortable to you a year ago is no longer comfortable, and what you imagined would never be comfortable or easy, now is enjoyable and natural! Once you adopt new, healthy, liberating habits into your life and embark on your long-dreamed-of adventures, you will inspire and become an example of hope to those around you who may be ready to "give up" on their dreams.

Daily Workout Summary -UPPER-BODY EXERCISES

Exercise 1: Biceps--Curl

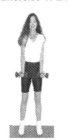 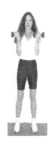

Exercise 2: Biceps-Hammer Curl

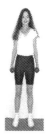 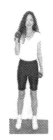

Exercise 3: Shoulders-Side Raise

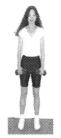 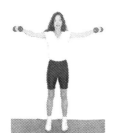

Exercise 4: Shoulders-Overhead Press

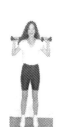 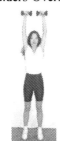

Exercise 5: Back-Bent Lift

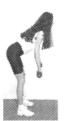 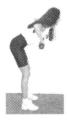

Exercise 6: Back-Upright Row

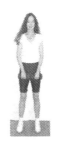 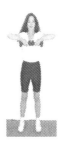

Exercise 7: Triceps-Extensions

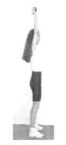 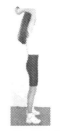

Exercise 8: Triceps-Pushback

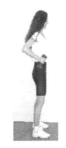 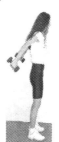

Exercise 9: Chest-Flye

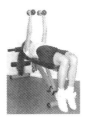

Exercise 10: Chest-Bench Press

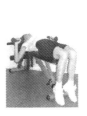 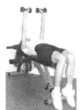

LOWER-BODY EXERCISES

Exercise 1: Calves-Straight-Toe Raise

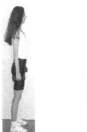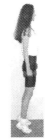

Exercise 2: Calves-Angled-Out-Toe Raise

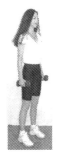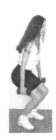

Exercise 3: Quadriceps/Glut-Squat

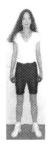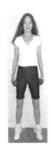

Exercise 4: Quadriceps/Glut-Squat
(Repeat of Exercise 3)

Exercise 5: Quadriceps--Extension

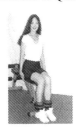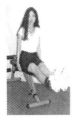

Exercise 6: Hamstring-Curls

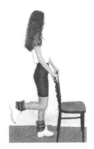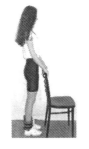

Exercise 7: Hamstring-Lunge

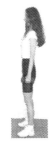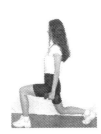

Exercise 8: Abdominal-Leg Lowering

Exercise 9: Abdominal-Crunch

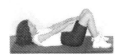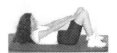

Exercise 10: Abdominal-Alternate Twist

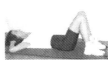

Alternate legs & arms.

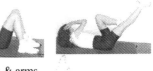

Printed in the United States
85193LV00001B/171-250/A

9 780979 745904